GOOD HOUSEKEEPING

Good Food for
DIABETICS

GOOD HOUSEKEEPING

Good Food for DIABETICS

THEODORA FITZGIBBON

Ebury Press London

Published by Ebury Press
Division of The National Magazine Company Ltd
Colquhoun House
27–37 Broadwick Street
London W1V 1FR

First impression 1988

ISBN 0 85223 629 8

Senior editors Veronica Sperling and Susie Ward
Editor Barbara Croxford
Design Bridgewater Associates
Photography Tim Imrie
Stylist Marie Jacques
Illustrator Annie Ellis
Cookery Janet Smith

Filmset by Advanced Filmsetters (Glasgow) Ltd
Printed and bound in Hong Kong by
Wing King Tong Co Ltd

CONTENTS

FOREWORD

My father became a diabetic in the early 1930's, when the treatment was very different from today; much sterner and more difficult for an active man to cope with. Several other members of my family are also diabetics so, you might think, I should be used to it.

However, when I became a diabetic some 20 years ago, I experienced a sense of shock and, to begin with, bewilderment. The leaflets one was given, about foods one could eat in limited quantities and those one couldn't, seemed very restricting. Yet, with a little forethought and common sense, as well as a reasonable knowledge of food, it is easily possible to enjoy a healthy, varied and excellent diet.

The key word is balance, which is why it makes such a very good title for the British Diabetic Association's magazine. I write about food all the time, not only in the thirty or so books I have had published, but also weekly, in a national newspaper. I have had to entertain quite a bit, yet never ever in all the meals I have prepared has any guest of mine been even slightly conscious that they were eating a diabetic diet. Such a diet is, in fact, a very healthy one. For today, we all know how inadequate sugar is in real food value, merely giving energy and promoting dental caries, whereas the natural fruit sugar, when taken with the whole fruit, pulp, juice and fibre, is much more healthful and is accompanied by valuable minerals and vitamins.

Fibre is important in all healthy diets and especially in the diabetic one, and brown breads and cakes are widely sought after by non-diabetics the world over; again, I stress that, if taken as a part of a balanced diet, they do no harm. All diabetics have to take a fairly large quota of carbohydrate, adjusted to their need, in their daily diet. I can assure you that, since becoming diabetic, I have never felt better or kept at such a steady weight, not too heavy for my build.

Travelling can be difficult, but always take with you some brown bread sandwiches, in case of flight or other delays, you get very used to it. My husband (a non-diabetic) insists on having his too! Having an appetising source of carbohydrate to hand prevents stress and worry, both of which are bad for diabetics.

Another important point, it really is vital to look at the fine print on food labels in shops. Nowadays, some quite unusual foods have sugar included in the ingredients, even ones we tend to think of as savoury, like some soy sauces. If the sugar is listed as being very small in amount, usually shown by being near the end of the list, then a little, occasionally taken, isn't too bad. However, generally speaking, it is safest to avoid such products and to choose those without the sugar. In many cases, sugar doesn't really improve the flavour anyway.

The recipes given in this book are those I use all the time, both for the family and entertaining, and I hope you enjoy them as much as we do.

THEODORA FITZGIBBON

INTRODUCTION

WHAT IS DIABETES?

DIABETES (*diabetes mellitus*) is a disorder characterised by raised blood glucose (blood sugar) levels known as hyperglycaemia.

Normal blood glucose levels are between 3.5 mmols per litre (65 mg per 100 ml) and 8 mmols per litre (145 mg per 100 ml). In the case of diabetes mellitus the level of glucose in the blood exceeds 8 mmols per litre (145 mg per 100 ml).

Blood glucose is the final breakdown product of carbohydrates (starches and sugars) present in our food after it has been fully digested and absorbed. It is the simplest form of sugar and used by the body as a primary source of energy. Levels of glucose in the blood are controlled by insulin, produced by the pancreas (a gland situated near the liver). Insulin is the hormone which instructs the cells to take up the blood glucose for energy production. In the diabetic, either no or insufficient insulin is being produced by the pancreas or the insulin produced cannot be used effectively.

If glucose is unable to enter the cells then levels in the blood begin to rise. The glucose will begin to spill out into the urine and can be detected by a simple urine test. Thirst and the passing of more urine than normal are early symptoms. Unexpected weight loss, blurring of eyesight and cramps in the legs can occur.

There are a number of ways of treating diabetes, including sensible eating.

1 If no insulin, or not enough, is being produced then daily injections of insulin are necessary. These might be once, twice or more times a day.

Insulin dependent diabetics (IDDM) are predominantly those who have developed the disorder when young (juvenile onset diabetes). They balance out their insulin with their dietary carbohydrate intake.

2 Non-insulin dependent diabetics (NIDDM) produce some insulin but the supply is inadequate. This is normally developed by mature people and is termed 'maturity onset diabetes'. Hypoglycaemic tablets (i.e. tablets which reduce levels of blood glucose, either by increasing insulin output by the pancreas or increasing the cells' ability to take up glucose), may be prescribed, together with a careful diet.

3 In other cases where some insulin is being produced, very careful attention to diet may be all that is needed.

Adults who are seriously overweight are more at risk of developing non-insulin dependent diabetes than those who are not so overweight. In such cases a balanced diet aimed at reducing weight may be all that is needed.

WHAT KIND OF DIET?

EATING A PROPERLY BALANCED DIET is important for everyone—diabetics and non-diabetics alike. The difference with diabetics is that it is very important to follow the diet in order to keep the disorder under control. To do this they normally have their diet tailored to their own individual needs by a qualified dietitian. Often this advice has so improved an individual's overall eating pattern that they feel far healthier than they ever did before. In fact, it may come as a pleasant surprise to some people just how varied and interesting meals can be which is well demonstrated by the recipes in this book.

What is meant by a properly balanced diet is the combination of carbohydrates, proteins and fats in such a way that sufficient energy, body-building materials, vitamins and minerals are eaten.

CARBOHYDRATES

Starchy carbohydrate foods that are high in fibre (e.g. unrefined cereals such as wholemeal flour, wholemeal bread, brown rice, whole grain breakfast cereals, plus pulses, vegetables and fruit) are digested more slowly than refined carbohydrate foods such as white flour, white rice, etc. This means that blood glucose levels do not rise so fast or so high and better control is maintained.

Carbohydrates to be avoided are table sugar, glucose, dextrose, corn syrup and honey, (known as simple sugars) and foods high in added sugar such as jam, sweets, puddings, cakes, biscuits, sugary, soft and fizzy drinks. Some simple sugars occur in commercial products such as digestive biscuits and baked beans. As these are in combination with unrefined starchy carbohydrates, there is a place for such products in the diet. There are particular occasions when simple sugars *are* called for—see HYPOGLYCAEMIA and EXERCISE.

EXCHANGES

Insulin dependent diabetics calculate carbohydrate using carbohydrate exchanges: 1 exchange (1 portion, 1 unit, or 1 line) = 10 grams carbohydrate.

Carbohydrate containing foods such as 1 apple, 1 small slice of bread or 1 small potato (weighing 50 grams/2 oz) each contain 10 grams of carbohydrate (i.e. 1 exchange). Using exchanges enables an individual to swap foods (using charts such as the one on page 10) and therefore extend the range of carbohydrate containing foods they can eat. The dietitian calculates the number and distribution of exchanges tailored to an individual's normal daily intake. This balance of insulin with food intake, enables insulin dependent diabetics to live normal and healthy lives.

ALTERNATIVE SWEETENERS

Alternative sweeteners such as artificial sweeteners (check that the crystal kinds do not have any added sugar), fructose (a fruit sugar that is digested in a different way from ordinary sugar), and sorbitol are available. Fructose is used in some of the recipes in this book. It is recommended that no more than 25 grams (1 oz) of fructose is eaten in any one day. Sorbitol is used commercially but has a laxative effect if eaten in any quantity. Both fructose and sorbitol have the same amount of energy (kcals/kJ) as ordinary sugar.

PROTEIN

Foods such as meat, poultry, fish, eggs, milk and cheese are main sources of protein and do not contribute any carbohydrate to the diet. Some of them, however, are high in fat and should be eaten in moderation. Lean meat, poultry and fish, together with fat-reduced milks and milk products should be chosen instead of high fat products. Oily fish such as herrings, kippers, salmon, etc., should be included because their oils have been found to be very beneficial in the prevention of heart disease.

MAIN DIETARY RECOMMENDATIONS

The main dietary recommendations are as follows:

▮ Match your energy intake (calories/kilojoules) to your individual requirements to maintain ideal weight. Lose weight if you are overweight.

▮ At *least half* the energy (calories/kilojoules) should come from starchy carbohydrates, particularly unrefined carbohydrates which are higher in fibre than refined products.

▮ Rapidly digested (refined) carbohydrates should only be taken in small amounts as part of a mixed fibre-rich meal.

▮ About one third of total energy intake (calories/kilojoules) should come from fat. Choose vegetable fats and oils.

ALCOHOL

Some alcoholic drinks contain carbohydrate. Obviously sweet drinks such as sweet sherries, sweet wines, sweet vermouths and liqueurs are to be avoided. Beer, stouts and lager also contain some carbohydrate so should only be drunk in moderation. Special diabetic beers (such as Diat) have just the same amount of energy (calories/kilojoules—kcals/kJ) as ordinary beers and often contain more alcohol! They do not have any advantages over ordinary beers.

No more than three alcoholic drinks should be taken in any one day (one drink is equivalent to 300 ml ($\frac{1}{2}$ pint) beer, cider or lager, one measure of spirits, one glass of wine, one small glass of sherry), and should be taken at the same time as food.

One drink would add approximately 100 kcals/418 kJ to the diet, so this should be taken into consideration, particularly by those on a weight reducing diet.

If drinking spirits (e.g. gin, whisky, vodka, etc) then choose a low calorie mixer such as water, low calorie tonic or ginger ale.

Insulin dependent diabetics should not eat less carbohydrate food to compensate for the carbohydrate in an alcoholic drink.

IT IS PARTICULARLY IMPORTANT THAT DIABETICS DO NOT DRINK AND DRIVE. Apart from alcohol's effect on the brain it also changes the way the liver produces glucose and it is possible to have a 'hypo' attack (see HYPOGLYCAEMIA on page 10). The symptoms of a 'hypo' are similar to drunkeness, so if a diabetic has been drinking alcohol, it may be extremely difficult for others to tell whether a true 'hypo' attack is occurring or not.

WHEN TO EAT

Just as important as the actual nutrients themselves is the timing of meals through the day. Three smallish meals, rather than fewer heavy meals, with large gaps in between, enables a better distribution of carbohydrate intake. It avoids either overloading the body with glucose (resulting in hyperglycaemia), or starving the body of glucose (hypoglycaemia).

Insulin dependent diabetics often require an in-between-meal snack to prevent a severe drop in their blood glucose as the insulin continues to work. The menu overleaf gives a good idea of a day's balanced eating—the light meal and main meal can be interchanged.

SUGGESTED MENU

	CHO grams	kcals/kJ
BREAKFAST		
40 g (1½ oz) Muesli, unsweetened with	30	150/630
1 Apple, grated into the muesli	10	50/210
200 ml (⅓ pint) Skimmed milk	10	65/260
Tea/Coffee		
MIDMORNING		
1 Digestive biscuit	10	70/295
Tea/Coffee		
LIGHT MEAL		
Leek and oatmeal soup	15	210/880
2 Thin large slices wholemeal bread	30	120/500
75 g (3 oz) Hummus	15	135/565
Green salad with French dressing	—	130/545
1 Small banana	10	40/165
MID-AFTERNOON		
1 Wholemeal apple scone	15	130/545
Tea/Coffee		
MAIN MEAL		
Lamb and courgette kebabs	—	230/960
175 g (6 oz) Boiled brown rice	50	210/880
100 g (4 oz) Carrots	—	20/85
Dessert—Apricot and orange coupe	20	105/440
BED-TIME		
200 ml (⅓ pint) Skimmed milk drink	10	65/270
1 Crunchy peanut butter biscuit	10	120/500
Daily skimmed milk allowance for teas and coffees 200 ml (⅓ pint)	10	65/270
TOTAL	245	1915/8000

Note: The above provides an average day's intake for a moderately active woman. It is not suitable for someone who is on a weight reducing diet. Skimmed milk has been assumed in the calculations, if you use semi-skimmed milk the total will be 2010/8415; whole milk 2105/8815.

HYPOGLYCAEMIA

Hypoglycaemia means low blood sugar which can be experienced by insulin dependent diabetics as well as those on hypoglaemic tablets. It can be brought on by not eating the right amount of carbohydrate at the right time, so that the levels of blood glucose drop below normal (3.5 mmols per litre or 65 mg per 100 ml).

The diabetic suffering a hypoglycaemic attack can experience weakness, hunger, sweating, faintness, headache and mental confusion. It is important that they take a rapidly absorbed form of carbohydrate such as sugar or glucose and are advised to always carry either sugar lumps or glucose tablets with them.

EXERCISE

Exercise plays an important part of the diabetic's life. It improves one's general well-being as well as making the insulin more effective—the body cells are able to take up the blood glucose more efficiently.

Extra carbohydrate foods may be required prior to, during, and after bouts of exercise. The amount of carbohydrate will depend on the type of exercise, but between 10–40 grams is a general rule. Before exercise choose a mixed carbohydrate food such as digestive biscuits. After exercise, eat some starchy carbohydrate, such as a wholemeal sandwich. It may, or may not be necessary to take some carbohydrate during the exercise. If it is necessary, take an easily absorbed form such as glucose tablets or carbohydrate containing drink.

WHAT TO DO WHEN ILL

WHEN UNWELL A LOSS OF APPETITE means that it is difficult to eat normally. It is important to continue taking insulin or tablets as usual and indeed the amount required may even be more than usual. The dose must be balanced by the usual amount of carbohydrate but it may be easier to take it in liquid form such as in milky or other sweetened drinks. Icecream, custard, rice pudding and fruit yogurts sweetened with ordinary sugar or honey are acceptable at this time.

GENERAL ADVICE FOR ALL DIABETICS

1 Keep to your diet
2 If you make changes in your diet or insulin dose inform your doctor or dietitian when you next see them
3 Visit your doctor or diabetic clinic regularly for check ups

4 Diabetes can affect your blood vessels so it is important that

▢ you look after your feet and have them checked by a chiropodist periodically. Report any sore places on your feet immediately

▢ your eyes are examined every year

▢ you have your blood pressure measured every year

THE BRITISH DIABETIC ASSOCIATION

THIS IS A NON-PROFIT MAKING ORGANISATION formed in 1934 by patients, doctors, scientists and ancillary workers involved in the treatment of diabetes. It provides help and advice to diabetics and promotes research into diabetes.

The Association produces the diabetic magazine 'BALANCE', together with very informative leaflets on diabetes and driving, pregnancy and other issues.

It has over 300 local groups nationwide where members get together for regular meetings and fund-raising events.

Their address is:
The British Diabetic Association
10 Queen Anne Street
London W1M 0BD
Tel. 01-323 1531

FIRST COURSES

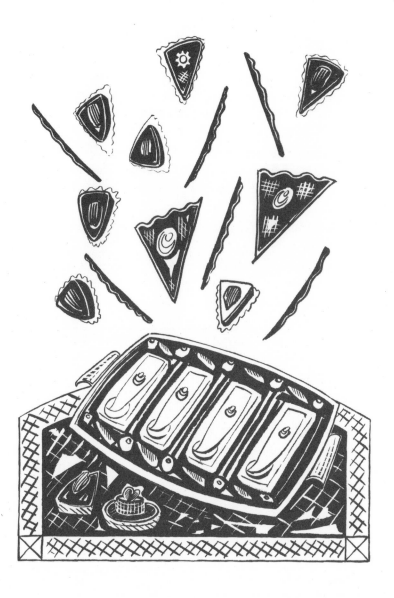

THE FIRST COURSE is a kind of curtain-raiser to the dinner, so what is to follow must be taken into account if the meal is to be well balanced. You want to avoid a mousse-like beginning if the pudding is similar in appearance and texture; if the main course is fairly heavy, then the first course should be light and vice versa.

Do not serve a soup, followed by a casserole-type dish. Avoid having cream in the first course, then a main course with a cream sauce, followed by a creamy pudding. In fact, the courses should stimulate the palate by their diversity from one another. What is needed is not only a change of taste but a difference in texture and colour too. First decide on your main course; then build around it.

See also Quick Meals on page 30, which include some egg dishes, Pasta, Rice and Pulses on page 84 and also Salads and Vegetables on page 96.

Courgette or Cucumber and Cheese Mousse

SERVE THIS ATTRACTIVE LIGHT MOUSSE with toast fingers or savoury biscuits.

INGREDIENTS
300 ml (½ pint) skimmed milk
1 bay leaf
sprig of parsley
sprig of tarragon
350 g (12 oz) curd or cottage cheese, drained
15 ml (1 tbsp) freshly squeezed lemon juice
225 g (8 oz) courgettes or cucumber, peeled and thinly sliced
150 ml (¼ pint) home-made Mayonnaise (see page 108)
150 ml (¼ pint) double cream
2 egg whites
20 g (¾ oz) powdered gelatine
fresh tarragon or burnet leaves, to garnish
SERVES 4 – 6

■ Put the milk, bay leaf and herbs into a saucepan and, just as the milk bubbles up, take off the heat and cover. Allow to infuse for 20 minutes.

■ Mix together the cheese and lemon juice. Strain the infused milk and reserve. Blanch the courgettes in boiling salted water for 2–3 minutes, then drain and cool.

■ Add the mayonnaise and milk to the cheese mixture, stirring well. Add the courgette to the mixture and liquidise. (If using cucumber, for a change, simply chop it further and stir in instead of liquidising.)

■ Whip the cream and egg whites sep-arately. Dissolve the gelatine in 45 ml (3 tbsp) hot water over a pan of simmering water. Add to the cheese and vegetable mixture, mixing well, then fold in the cream and egg whites.

■ Pour the mousse into a damp 1.4 litre (2½ pint) ring mould, if available. Chill until set. When set, turn out and garnish with fresh tarragon or burnet leaves, or a pattern of both.

4 SERVINGS		6 SERVINGS	
kcals	635	kcals	425
kJ	2656	kJ	1780
CHO	10 g	CHO	5 g
Fibre	0	Fibre	0

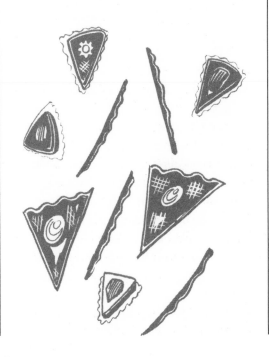

Liver Pâté

SERVED WITH TOAST, liver pâté makes a useful light lunch, with a soup first and fruit afterwards. Any liver can be used for this pâté but I think the best is duck or chicken liver. It is quick and simple to make.

INGREDIENTS
450 g (1 lb) liver
2 garlic cloves, skinned and crushed
small pinch of dried sage
small pinch of dried tarragon
75 ml ($\frac{1}{8}$ pint) red wine or consommé
1 egg yolk
salt and freshly ground black pepper
4 rashers bacon, derinded (optional)
1 bay leaf
SERVES 4 – 6

■ Mince the liver or put into a food processor until finely minced. Add the garlic, herbs and wine or consommé. Finally stir in the egg yolk and season to taste.

■ If using the bacon rashers, stretch them, by holding one end and running the flat of the blade of a heavy knife along the length. Put the bay leaf into the bottom of a lightly oiled ovenproof dish or loaf tin. Cover the base with the bacon rashers. If not using the rashers, it is important to oil the dish or tin.

■ Add the liver mixture. Place the dish or tin into another larger one containing enough hot water to come half way up the sides of the inner one. Cover the pâté with foil.

■ Bake at 180°C (350°F) mark 4 for about 1 hour. Leave to cool, but not in the refrigerator. When cool, press the pâté. To do this, cover the pâté with a small wooden board, which fits the dish or tin. Put weights or heavy cans of food on top and leave until completely cold. This pâté will keep for a week in a really cool larder. Otherwise, cover with foil and store in the least cool part of the refrigerator. It will be spoiled if frozen.

4 SERVINGS		6 SERVINGS	
kcals	290	kcals	195
kJ	1215	kJ	810
CHO	Negligible	CHO	Negligible
Fibre	0	Fibre	0

Eggs Stuffed with Caviare (lumpfish roe)

A VERY QUICK AND EASY first course which can be made ahead of time.

INGREDIENTS
4 eggs, size 3, boiled for 12 minutes and soaked in cold water
30 ml (2 tbsp) natural yogurt
few drops of Tabasco or Chilli sherry relish (see page 147)
salt and freshly ground black pepper
150 g (5 oz) jar of black or red lumpfish roe
few crisp lettuce leaves or little watercress
lemon wedges, to serve
SERVES 4

■ Refrigerate the hard-boiled eggs. When chilled, slice in half lengthways. With a small spoon, carefully take out the yolks and put them into a medium bowl. Mash thoroughly.

▌ Mix in the yogurt, using just enough to achieve a soft but not sloppy mixture. Continue vigorous stirring with a fork until smooth, adding the Tabasco or Chilli sherry relish, a few drops at a time, until the right balance of flavour is obtained. Add the seasoning, but do not add too much salt as the caviare is salty.

▌ Take a small slice off the rounded bottoms of the egg halves so that they stand evenly. Refill them with the mixture and arrange on a serving plate, allowing 2 halves per person. Just before serving, top each with a spoonful of caviare and serve with lettuce and a lemon wedge on each plate.

4 SERVINGS	
kcals	167
kJ	699
CHO	Negligible
Fibre	0

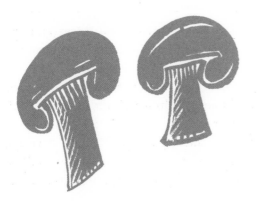

Mushrooms with Pâté in Consommé

ANOTHER VERY QUICK AND EASY first course, provided you have some pâté, either fresh or canned, in the house, as well as consommé and some good sized mushrooms. It is delicious and most filling.

INGREDIENTS
6 slices of pâté
6 medium to large mushrooms, wiped, stalks removed
salt
15 ml (1 tbsp) freshly squeezed lemon juice
nut of butter or margarine
300 ml ($\frac{1}{2}$ pint) consommé
SERVES 6

▌ Put a thick slice of pâté into 6 cocotte pots, just covering the bottom. Put the mushrooms in a saucepan containing enough boiling salted water to cover with the lemon juice and butter added. Cover the liquid surface with greaseproof paper or foil to exclude the air and poach for 5 minutes.

▌ Drain the mushrooms and pat dry, reserving the cooking liquid as it makes an ingredient for stock.

▌ When cool, put a mushroom on top of each slice of pâté. Pour over enough consommé to cover well. Place in the refrigerator to set. Serve chilled with slices of toast.

6 SERVINGS	
kcals	230
kJ	955
CHO	0
Fibre	2

Terrine aux Herbes

6 SERVINGS		8 SERVINGS	
kcals	380	kcals	285
kJ	1580	kJ	1185
CHO	5 g	CHO	Negligible
Fibre	0	Fibre	0

THIS TERRINE LOOKS PRETTY when cut, with the fresh green herbs marbling the meats. If you have to use dried herbs, halve the quantity.

INGREDIENTS

450 g (1 lb) spinach, washed
salt
450 g (1 lb) minced pork or sausagemeat
100 g (4 oz) cooked ham, diced
100 g (4 oz) unsmoked bacon, diced
2 garlic cloves, skinned and finely chopped
2 small onions, skinned and finely chopped
30 ml (2 tbsp) finely chopped fresh parsley
10 ml (2 tsp) finely chopped fresh basil
pinch of chervil
pinch of rosemary
pinch of cayenne pepper
pinch of freshly grated nutmeg
2 eggs, beaten
strips of pork fat or streaky bacon

SERVES 6 – 8

■ Cook the spinach in a saucepan with 30–45 ml (2–3 tbsp) water and a little salt for 5 minutes only. Drain and squeeze well to remove the liquid. Chop the spinach.

■ Mix the spinach with the minced pork or sausagemeat. Mix the ham and bacon with the garlic, onions and herbs. Mix all the ingredients together, season well and stir in the eggs.

■ Press the mixture into a lightly greased terrine dish. Cover with the pork or bacon strips, then with foil and the lid. Cook at 180°C (350°F) mark 4 for about 1½– 2 hours. Cool, turn out and slice to serve.

Spinach and Sardine Pâté

SO LIGHT AND DELICATE, this pâté could almost be called a mousse. It makes an excellent first course, or a main course for a light lunch. A very successful cold buffet dish too.

INGREDIENTS

15 ml (3 tsp) powdered gelatine
100 g (4 oz) full fat soft cheese or cottage cheese
175 g (6 oz) cooked spinach, either fresh or frozen, well drained
15 ml (1 tbsp) freshly squeezed lemon juice
four 120 g (4½ oz) cans sardines in oil, drained
salt and freshly ground black pepper
freshly grated nutmeg
To garnish
1 hard-boiled egg, sliced
burnet leaves

SERVES 8

■ Put 45 ml (3 tbsp) hot water and the gelatine into a liquidiser or food processor and blend on high for about 30 seconds. Add the cheese, in pieces, cover and blend again for about 1 minute until well creamed.

■ Add the spinach in batches, covering and blending until smoothly puréed together with no white showing. Pour in the

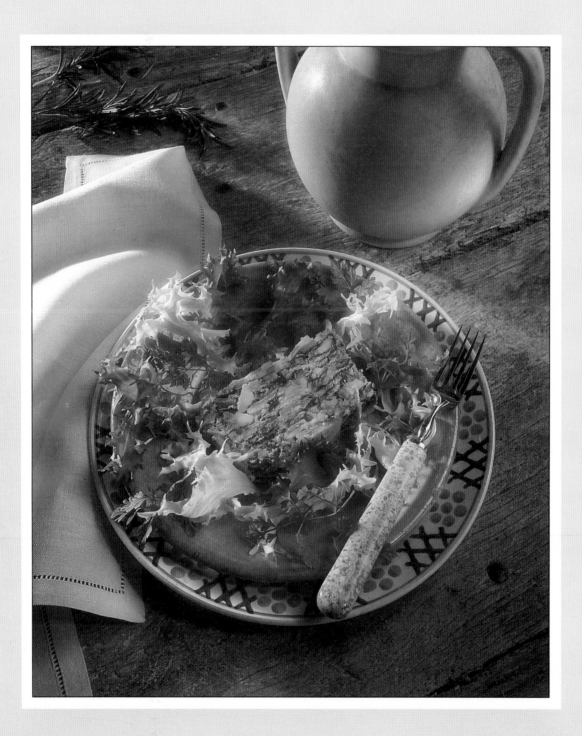

Terrine aux Herbes (opposite)

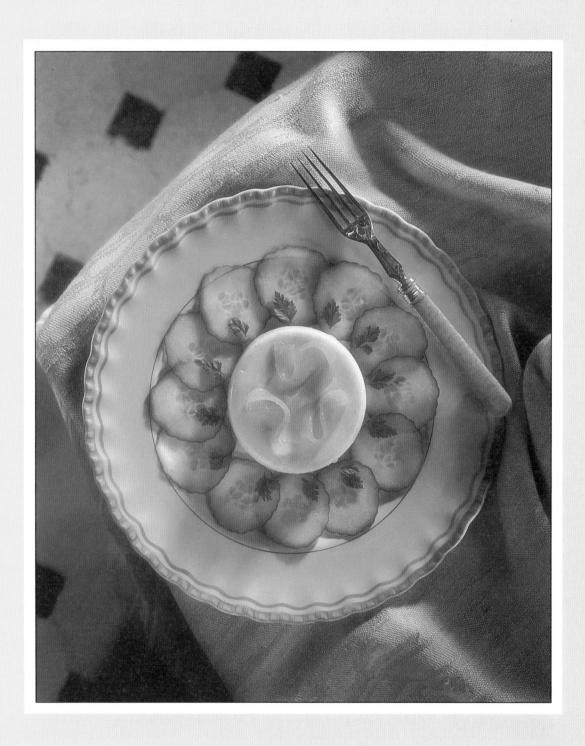

Smoked Salmon Mousses (page 18)

lemon juice while blending, then add the sardines. Blend very thoroughly, then season to taste, adding a pinch of nutmeg.

■ Wet a 1 litre (2 pint) mould, spoon in the mixture, or fill individual pots. Cover and chill for about 2–3 hours until well set. Unmould and garnish with egg slices and burnet leaves. Chill until serving time.

WITH LOW-FAT CHEESE		WITH HIGH-FAT CHEESE	
kcals	155	kcals	195
kJ	645	kJ	825
CHO	Negligible	CHO	Negligible
Fibre	1.5	Fibre	1.5

Mushrooms Stuffed with Blue Cheese

YOU NEED A GOOD BLUE CHEESE for this, such as Stilton or Gorgonzola.

INGREDIENTS
450 g (1 lb) medium open mushrooms, wiped, stalks removed
15 ml (1 tbsp) freshly squeezed lemon juice
nut of butter or margarine
175 g (6 oz) blue cheese
100 g (4 oz) cottage cheese
50 g (2 oz) walnuts, finely chopped
30 ml (2 tbsp) red wine
60 ml (4 tbsp) finely chopped fresh parsley
SERVES 4 – 6

■ Put the mushrooms in a saucepan of boiling salted water with the lemon juice and butter added. Cover the liquid surface with greaseproof paper or foil to exclude the air and poach for not more than 5 minutes. Drain the mushrooms, pat dry and chill. Keep the salted water for stock.

■ Meanwhile, mix together the blue and cottage cheeses in a bowl until the mixture is perfectly smooth. (If you have one, use a food processor for this.) Add the walnuts, red wine and 30 ml (2 tbsp) of the chopped parsley. Continue mixing or processing until evenly mixed.

■ Arrange the mushrooms on a large dish, hollow cups uppermost, and fill the centres with the mixture, piping it on if wished. Garnish with the remainder of the parsley and serve chilled. They are excellent, too, with Yogurt spiced sauce (see page 113).

4 SERVINGS		6 SERVINGS	
kcals	275	kcals	185
kJ	1150	kJ	775
CHO	Negligible	CHO	Negligible
Fibre	4 g	Fibre	3 g

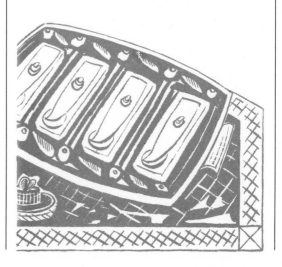

Tuna Fish Pâté

THIS IS REALLY AN EMERGENCY first course from the store cupboard, but good none the less. The amount of butter can be reduced and more cottage cheese used, if preferred.

INGREDIENTS

two 175 g (6 oz) cans of tuna fish, drained
175 g (6 oz) butter
175 g (6 oz) cottage cheese
15 ml (1 tbsp) finely chopped fresh parsley
15 ml (1 tbsp) finely chopped fresh chives
salt and freshly ground black pepper
few drops of Tabasco sauce or Chilli sherry relish (see page 147)
10 ml (2 tsp) freshly squeezed lemon juice
30 ml (2 tbsp) French capers, drained

SERVES 6

■ Mix the tuna fish with the butter and cottage cheese in a bowl. Add the parsley and chives, season to taste, then add the Tabasco or Chilli sherry relish and lemon juice to taste. Lastly, mix in the capers.

■ Shape the pâté into an oblong or round and serve surrounded with fresh raw vegetables and slices of toast.

6 SERVINGS	
kcals	330
kJ	1380
CHO	Negligible
Fibre	0

Smoked Salmon Mousse

A RECIPE WHICH HAS the advantage of making a little smoked salmon go a surprisingly long way. It can be made using the trimmings left from the slicing of a smoked salmon and these can be bought, reasonably cheaply, at most good fish shops. It is best to use a liquidiser or food processor, if you have one.

INGREDIENTS

5 ml (1 tsp) aspic powder or 2.5 ml ($\frac{1}{2}$ tsp) powdered gelatine
225 g (8 oz) cottage cheese or curd cheese
50 g (2 oz) smoked salmon trimmings
squeeze of fresh lemon juice
few drops of Tabasco sauce or pinch of cayenne pepper
lettuce leaves, to serve
smoked salmon trimmings, to garnish

SERVES 4 – 6

■ Put 300 ml ($\frac{1}{2}$ pint) boiling water into a liquidiser or food processor, add the aspic powder or gelatine and blend for 30 seconds. Add all the remaining ingredients and blend for about 1 minute.

■ Taste for seasoning, adjust if needed. Put at once into a dish or individual dishes and chill. It will set very quickly, within an hour. Unmould and serve on a bed of lettuce leaves, garnished with smoked salmon trimmings.

4 SERVINGS		6 SERVINGS	
kcals	75	kcals	50
kJ	315	kJ	210
CHO	Negligible	CHO	Negligible
Fibre	0	Fibre	0

BONED KIPPERS, smoked mackerel or smoked trout can also be used instead of smoked salmon, but use double the fish.

Vegetable and Herb Pâté

THIS VERY ATTRACTIVE DISH makes a good summer first course or a light lunch, with cheese and fresh fruit afterwards. This pâté can be made in advance a day ahead of time.

INGREDIENTS

225 g (8 oz) spinach, trimmed of stalks and washed

450 g (1 lb) courgettes, grated, or mushrooms, finely chopped

salt and freshly ground black pepper

50 g (2 oz) butter

450 g (1 lb) young carrots, scraped and finely grated

225 g (8 oz) sieved cottage cheese or low-fat curd cheese

4 eggs, size 4, beaten

30 ml (2 tbsp) natural yogurt

pinch of dry mustard powder

15 ml (1 tbsp) chopped fresh parsley

15 ml (1 tbsp) chopped fresh chives

cucumber slices, to garnish

SERVES 6 – 8

▪ Steam the spinach for 2 minutes only and drain well. Line the sides and base of a 1 kg (2 lb) loaf tin with non-stick paper. Line the tin with the spinach leaves and put aside.

▪ Put the grated courgettes in a colander, sprinkle with salt and leave for 30 minutes. Drain off any liquid and pat dry with absorbent kitchen paper.

▪ While the courgettes are marinating, melt the butter in a pan and cook the carrots until tender but do not allow them to colour. Add the courgettes, stirring continuously, until a soft purée is formed. Allow to cool.

▪ Mix the cottage cheese into the eggs with the yogurt, mustard powder and herbs, together with the purée of carrot and courgette. Liquidise if preferred. Season well to taste.

▪ Pour the mixture into the spinach-lined tin, being careful not to disturb the spinach leaves, then stand in a larger tin with hot water, up to 2.5 cm (1 inch) deep.

▪ Cook at 180°C (350°F) mark 4 for $1\frac{1}{4}$ hours or until firm to the touch. Cool in the tin. Carefully run a thin, sharp knife around the edges, put the inverted serving dish on top, reverse quickly, with a slight shake to unmould, if needed. Peel off any paper adhering and chill to firm up, but do not serve the pâté too cold. Garnish with sliced cucumber or other raw vegetables around the edges. Cut into slices to serve.

6 SERVINGS		8 SERVINGS	
kcals	200	kcals	150
kJ	845	kJ	635
CHO	10 g	CHO	5 g
Fibre	2 g	Fibre	2 g

SOUPS

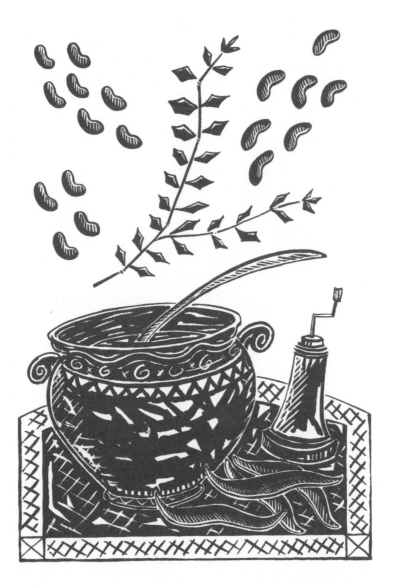

ALL KINDS OF SOUPS are an invaluable part of the diabetic's diet. Clear soups, which have no carbohydrate or calories, are a free 'extra' and these can be either hot or cold. They are good 'fillers' to stem hunger and have the added advantage of being cool on a hot day or deliciously warming on a cold one. All soups are better made with home-made stock, so don't throw away leftover bones of either meat or poultry or, for that matter, fish.

'Main course' soups are very good for those living alone, for they can be added to and used for light lunches. However, if keeping soups, either in the refrigerator or a cool larder, when reheating them, be sure that they are brought absolutely to the boil and kept at a boil for at least 5 minutes.

Soups are a very good way of keeping up your carbohydrate balance if you are ill and not tempted by more usual food.

Avocado Soup

THIS RECIPE MAKES AN AVOCADO go a long way and the softer, sometimes cheaper, ones can be used. A liquidiser is essential to make this soup.

INGREDIENTS
flesh of 2 ripe avocados
1 shallot or very small onion, skinned
900 ml (1½ pints) chicken stock
salt and freshly ground black pepper
300 ml (½ pint) creamy milk
150 ml (¼ pint) natural yogurt or cream
squeeze of fresh lemon juice
To garnish
thin slices of avocado
parsley
SERVES 6

■ Put the flesh of the avocados, the shallot, chicken stock and seasoning into a liquidiser and blend at high speed for 40 seconds.

■ Add the creamy milk, yogurt and lemon juice. Cover and blend again, taste for seasoning, adding a little more stock if too thick. Put the covered container in the refrigerator.

■ Just before serving, for the garnish cut thin slices of avocado and liberally squeeze lemon juice on both sides to prevent them from going brown. Blend the soup for a few seconds, add the garnish and immediately serve cold.

6 SERVINGS	
kcals	190
kJ	795
CHO	5 g
Fibre	1 g

Courgette Soup

MANY STOCK CUBES are rather salty, although there are some cubes with very little salt content available at health food shops.

INGREDIENTS
400 ml (14 fl oz) home-made chicken stock or use a chicken stock cube
3 medium courgettes, sliced
2 medium onions, skinned and chopped
1 garlic clove, skinned and sliced
225 ml (8 fl oz) mayonnaise or natural yogurt
5 ml (1 tsp) freshly squeezed lemon juice
1.25 ml (¼ tsp) freshly grated nutmeg
1.25 ml (¼ tsp) salt
1 lemon, very thinly sliced, to garnish
SERVES 4

■ Put the chicken stock, courgettes, onions and garlic into a saucepan. Bring to the boil, cover and simmer for 10 minutes or until the vegetables are tender.

■ Cool, then liquidise in batches until smooth and uniform in texture. Pour the soup into a large bowl, then stir in the remaining ingredients. Cover and chill overnight. Serve cold, garnishing with thinly cut lemon slices.

4 SERVINGS	
kcals	60
kJ	250
CHO	10 g
Fibre	0

Fish Soup

THIS MAKES THE MOST WARMING and good fish soup-stew. If liked, serve with bread croûtons, fried in oil with crushed garlic.

INGREDIENTS

900 g (2 lb) assorted white fish fillets, such as haddock or cod, and a firm one, such as monkfish if available, skinned

little flour

salt and freshly ground black pepper

610 ml (generous 1 pint) fish stock (see page 47)

425 g (15 oz) can tomatoes

pinch of fennel seeds

pinch of basil

pinch of saffron (optional)

2 medium potatoes, peeled and cubed

Tabasco or Worcestershire sauce

chopped fresh parsley, to garnish

SERVES 6

■ Cube all the fish and roll in the flour, seasoned with salt and pepper. Put the fish stock into a large saucepan and add the firm fish. Bring to the boil, add the tomatoes and their juice, the herbs, saffron if using, and potatoes. Cook gently until the potatoes are tender.

■ Add the rest of the fish. Cook for no longer than 10–15 minutes, then taste and adjust the seasoning, if necessary. Add a few drops of Tabasco or Worcestershire sauce. Garnish thickly with chopped fresh parsley.

6 SERVINGS	
kcals	155
kJ	650
CHO	10 g
Fibre	1 g

Lentil Soup—Zuppa di Lenticchie

IF YOU HAVE A PRESSURE COOKER, the cooking time can be reduced to 30 minutes from the time it reaches full pressure.

INGREDIENTS

30 ml (2 tbsp) oil, preferably olive

2 rashers bacon, chopped

1 medium to large carrot, scraped and sliced

1–2 celery stalks with a few leaves, sliced

1 large onion, skinned and sliced

225 g (8 oz) brown or green lentils, soaked overnight

10 ml (2 tsp) whole coriander seeds or 5 ml (1 tsp) ground

15 ml (1 tbsp) chopped fresh parsley

1.1 litres (2 pints) stock or water, preferably ham stock

salt and freshly ground black pepper

SERVES 4

■ Heat the oil in a pan and fry the bacon, then very lightly sauté the carrot, celery and onion but on no account allow them to take colour. Add the lentils and their soaking water, the coriander, half the parsley and the stock.

■ Cover, bring to the boil and simmer for about 1½ hours, stirring from time to time; test for tenderness—they might need another 30 minutes.

■ When cooked, leave to cool, then reheat before serving. Taste for seasoning and garnish with the remaining parsley. (If salt is added before the lentils are cooked, it can make them hard.) Traditionally, this is a thick soup, but can be thinned with a little more stock.

4 SERVINGS	
kcals	305
kJ	1275
CHO	35 g
Fibre	8 g

VARIATION

IN ITALY, this soup is served with some of the sweet Italian sausages, the ones without fennel seeds. It is good with our sausages too, if they are first cooked until brown on the outside, then spread with a little mild mustard, chopped and added to the soup before serving. Allow about 2 small sausages per person.

Leek and Oatmeal Soup

THIS IS A VERY OLD traditional soup, known as *Brotchan Roy* in Irish. Not only is it delicious and easy to make, but it is also full of fibre!

INGREDIENTS
4–6 large leeks, washed and trimmed
25 g (1 oz) butter
1.4 litres (2½ pints) half milk and half chicken stock
60 ml (4 tbsp) rolled oats
salt and freshly ground black pepper
30 ml (2 tbsp) chopped fresh parsley
150 ml (¼ pint) single cream, to garnish
SERVES 6

▮ Leaving most of the fresher green parts on, chop the leeks into chunks about 2.5 cm (1 inch) long, then wash again if needed.

▮ Put the butter, milk and stock into a large saucepan over a medium heat. When boiling, add the oats and boil for 5 minutes, then add the leeks and season well. Cover and simmer gently for about 30 minutes.

▮ Add 15 ml (1 tbsp) of the chopped parsley and cook for 5 minutes more. Serve in bowls with a little cream in each and the remainder of the parsley sprinkled over.

6 SERVINGS	
kcals	210
kJ	880
CHO	15 g
Fibre	3 g

VARIATIONS

STREAKY BACON, cooked until really crisp, crushed with a rolling pin and scattered over, makes a pleasant addition.

Smoked Haddock and Leek Soup

POACH 350 g (12 oz) SMOKED HADDOCK or other smoked fish in milk to cover. Skin and remove any bones. Flake the fish into the soup at the same time the leeks are added. Adjust the seasoning to taste.

TWO SIMPLE SOUPS
WITH YOGURT

Chachik

THIS IS A TURKISH FIRST COURSE or soup, perfect on a summer's day. Chachik also makes a very good sauce to serve with cold fish, such as salmon or mackerel, and a good spoonful is delicious beside hot, buttery potatoes or in place of cream in a baked potato.

INGREDIENTS
1 garlic clove, cut
1 small to medium cucumber, peeled and grated or finely diced
salt
600 ml (1 pint) natural yogurt, chilled
15 ml (1 tbsp) finely chopped fresh mint, to garnish
SERVES 4

▮ Rub around each soup bowl with the cut garlic clove. Scatter the cucumber with a little salt, mix and marinate for 5 minutes.

▮ Mix the cucumber into the yogurt, then distribute the mixture into 4 bowls (in really hot weather, it is a good idea to chill the bowls first.) Garnish liberally with the mint. It really has to be fresh mint to get the right effect!

4 SERVINGS	
kcals	85
kJ	355
CHO	10 g
Fibre	0

Cold Yogurt Soup

THIS IS THE QUICKEST and easiest cold soup in the world. Simply beat together two 568 g (1 pint) cartons of chilled natural yogurt with about a third of the quantity of chilled plain tomato juice, adding a little salt to taste. It is best to use the plain, unseasoned tomato juice or the flavour of the yogurt will be lost.

This refreshing soup serves 4; but can be made for more by using extra yogurt and tomato juice. Garnish with prawns, cucumber cubes or courgettes, thinly sliced, all with a sprinkling of paprika.

4 SERVINGS	
kcals	170
kJ	710
CHO	20 g
Fibre	0

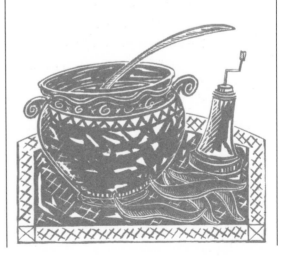

Tuscan Bean Soup

THE ADDITION OF SMOKED or fresh cooked, chopped sausages or pieces of cooked bacon will make this a very substantial meal.

INGREDIENTS

450 g (1 lb) dried white beans, soaked overnight, or two 450 g (1 lb) cans butter beans, drained
30 ml (2 tbsp) oil, preferably olive
2 rashers streaky bacon, chopped
1 large onion, skinned and sliced
1 garlic clove, skinned and crushed, or 2.5 ml (½ tsp) minced garlic
2 celery stalks or celery flakes, to taste
200 g (7 oz) can tomatoes
5 ml (1 tsp) dried oregano
salt and freshly ground black pepper
600 ml (1 pint) stock

SERVES 6 – 8

∎ If using dried beans, drain and put into a saucepan. Cover with fresh cold water, bring to the boil and discard the water. Cover again with fresh water, bring to the boil and simmer for about 1 hour.

∎ If using the canned beans, drain them of all liquid from the can, rinse in cold water and put into a saucepan, adding 600 ml (1 pint) water.

∎ Heat the oil in a saucepan and lightly fry the bacon. Add the onion and garlic and soften but do not brown. Add the celery, then the tomatoes and their juice.

∎ Stir the mixture into the beans. If using canned beans, stirring must be gentle to avoid breaking them up. Add the oregano and black pepper, then the stock. Bring back to the boil and simmer for 2 hours if using dried beans. If using canned beans, simmer for 30 minutes or until the celery is cooked. (If using a pressure cooker for the dried beans, the time at full pressure should be about 30 minutes. It is not advisable to use a pressure cooker for the canned beans as the canning has pressure cooked them already.) Taste and adjust the seasoning.

6 SERVINGS		8 SERVINGS	
kcals	295	kcals	220
kJ	1235	kJ	920
CHO	35 g	CHO	25 g
Fibre	20 g	Fibre	15 g

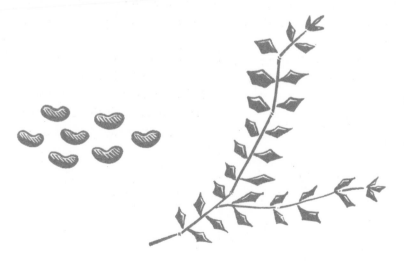

Red Pepper Soup

DO NOT USE too much cream for garnishing.

INGREDIENTS

2 medium red peppers, cored and deseeded
25 g (1 oz) butter or margarine
1 medium to large onion, skinned and sliced
600 ml (1 pint) chicken stock
1.25 ml ($\frac{1}{4}$ tsp) dried oregano
salt and freshly ground black pepper
30 ml (2 tbsp) plain flour
300 ml ($\frac{1}{2}$ pint) milk
cream, to garnish

SERVES 4

■ Finely slice and chop the peppers, keeping a few strips for garnish. Heat 15 g ($\frac{1}{2}$ oz) of the butter in a saucepan until foaming and fry the peppers and onion until soft but not browned. Add the chicken stock and oregano, season to taste, mix well and simmer for about 10–15 minutes. Purée in a liquidiser or mouli-legume.

■ Heat the rest of the butter in a saucepan, add the flour, mix well and cook for 1 minute. Take off the heat, gradually add the milk, stirring well. Heat, still stirring, until smooth and creamy.

■ Add the puréed pepper mixture. Reheat if serving hot, or chill. Garnish with pepper strips and cream.

4 SERVINGS	
kcals	105
kJ	440
CHO	10 g
Fibre	1 g

Lettuce Soup

SERVED HOT OR COLD, this makes a perfect first course which, if you have some lettuce in the garden, is cheap to make.

INGREDIENTS

2 large lettuces
25 g (1 oz) butter
6 spring onions, trimmed and chopped, or a handful of chopped chives
30 ml (2 tbsp) plain flour
900 ml (1$\frac{1}{2}$ pints) chicken stock
150 ml ($\frac{1}{4}$ pint) milk
pinch of fructose
pinch of freshly grated nutmeg
salt and freshly ground black pepper
cream or natural yogurt, to garnish
fried croûtons, to serve

SERVES 6

■ Remove any hard stalks from the lettuce, then cut into fine ribbons. Melt the butter in a saucepan and very lightly fry the lettuce and spring onions until soft but not coloured, stirring all the time.

■ Sprinkle over the flour and cook for 1 minute, then gradually add the stock, stirring well. When smooth and slightly thickened, add the milk, fructose and nutmeg and taste for seasoning. Simmer for about 10 minutes.

■ Either sieve or liquidise the soup. Garnish with a little cream or yogurt and serve the croûtons separately.

6 SERVINGS	
kcals	115
kJ	485
CHO	10 g
Fibre	2 g

Carrot and Orange Soup

TO MAKE THE ORANGE BUTTER, work grated orange rind into butter.

INGREDIENTS

450 g (1 lb) carrots, scraped and finely chopped
1 large onion, skinned and finely chopped
1.7 litres (3 pints) chicken stock
juice and grated rind of 2 small oranges
pinch of ground coriander
salt and freshly ground black pepper
30–45 ml (2–3 tbsp) cream or creamy milk, to garnish

SERVES ABOUT 6

■ Put the carrots and onion into a large saucepan and add the stock. Do not season yet, but bring to the boil and simmer until the carrots are quite soft.

■ Liquidise, return to the saucepan and add the juice of the oranges and the coriander. Heat through and taste for seasoning. Garnish with cream or creamy milk and serve with brown bread spread with orange butter.

6 SERVINGS	
kcals	35
kJ	145
CHO	5 g
Fibre	2 g

Scotch Broth

THIS EXCELLENT SATISFYING SOUP is indeed a meal in itself.

INGREDIENTS

2 knuckles of lamb or 1 boned neck
1.7 litres (3 pints) cold water
salt and freshly ground white pepper
1 large onion, skinned and sliced
3 large carrots, scraped and sliced
3 white turnips, peeled and sliced
1 bay leaf
about 65 g (2½ oz) pearl barley
chopped fresh parsley, to garnish

SERVES 6

■ Put the lamb knuckles or neck into a saucepan containing the cold water. Season, bring to the boil and simmer for 1–1½ hours until the meat is tender. Lift out and allow the stock to cool.

■ When the stock is cold and the fat has congealed on the surface, skim it away and make up the liquid to about 2.3 litres (4 pints) with water. Add the onion, carrots and turnips to the stock together with the bay leaf. Bring to the boil and simmer for about 30 minutes.

■ Taste for seasoning and add the pearl barley. Simmer for about 1 hour.

■ Meanwhile, defat and debone the meat, cut into bite sized pieces and add to the soup when the barley is cooked. Return to a simmer and sprinkle with parsley.

6 SERVINGS	
kcals	165
kJ	690
CHO	15 g
Fibre	4 g

Mushroom Soup

THIS SOUP, quite different from most mushroom soup recipes, is very fresh tasting with a lemony tang.

INGREDIENTS
15 ml (1 tbsp) oil, preferably sunflower
2 medium onions, skinned and finely chopped
450 g (1 lb) mushrooms, finely chopped
salt and freshly ground black pepper
900 ml (1½ pints) chicken stock
15 ml (1 tbsp) freshly squeezed lemon juice
pinch of freshly grated nutmeg
5–10 ml (1–2 tsp) mushroom ketchup (optional)
To garnish
chopped fresh parsley
thin lemon slices
SERVES 4

■ Heat the oil in a medium saucepan and very gently cook the onions until soft but not coloured. (This is easier if a lid is put on and the heat kept low.) When the onions are half cooked, add the mushrooms, turning them over well so that they mix with the onions and oil. If the contents of the saucepan appear to be getting too dry, add a little more oil as the cooking progresses, but be careful not to add too much.

■ When the mushrooms are just soft, season, add the stock and bring to the boil. Lower to a simmer and add the lemon juice, stirring well. Cover and simmer gently for 30–40 minutes.

■ Taste again for seasoning and adjust if needed. Add the nutmeg and mushroom ketchup if using, take off the heat and allow to cool slightly. Either liquidise or put through a food processor in batches. Reheat, pour into bowls and garnish with the parsley. Serve with thin slices of lemon sprinkled with chopped parsley.

4 SERVINGS	
kcals	50
kJ	210
CHO	Negligible
Fibre	4 g

French Onion Soup

THIS FAMOUS SOUP is really excellent and can be made easily in half an hour. Use the red wine for the authentic version.

INGREDIENTS
30 ml (2 tbsp) oil or 25 g (1 oz) butter
4 large onions, skinned and thinly sliced
pinch of fructose
salt and freshly ground black pepper
30 ml (2 tbsp) flour
1.7 litres (3 pints) beef stock, use cubes if necessary
150 ml (¼ pint) red wine (optional)
6 rounds of thick French bread or Vienna loaf
75 g (3 oz) cheese, grated
SERVES 6

■ Heat the oil in a large pan and cook the onions over a low heat, turning from time to time, until soft and just golden coloured. (Do not let the onions brown, as this can make them bitter.)

■ Add the fructose, pepper and a little salt, remembering that the cheese will be quite salty. Sprinkle over the flour and mix well. Gradually add the stock and wine if using, stirring until smooth and the soup has returned to the boil. Cover and simmer gently for about 20–25 minutes.

■ Meanwhile, dry out the bread or lightly toast it. Pour the soup into individual heatproof bowls, float the bread on top and sprinkle with cheese. Put the bowls under a hot grill, or into a hot oven, until the cheese is bubbling and slightly browned.

6 SERVINGS	
kcals	160
kJ	670
CHO	15 g
Fibre	2 g

Cucumber Soup

A VERY REFRESHING SOUP served cold in warm weather, but it can be served hot too.

INGREDIENTS
25 g (1 oz) butter
2 medium cucumbers, peeled and chopped
30 ml (2 tbsp) plain flour
1.1 litres (2 pints) chicken stock
1 small onion, skinned and sliced
300 ml (½ pint) creamy milk
salt and freshly ground white pepper
2 egg yolks and 30 ml (2 tbsp) cream (if serving hot)
chopped fresh chives or parsley, to garnish
SERVES 6

■ Melt the butter in a saucepan and soften the cucumber, but do not let it brown. Add the flour, then stir in the stock. Bring to the boil and simmer gently for about 20 minutes or until cooked.

■ Scald the onion in the milk, then combine both mixtures. Taste for seasoning. Either sieve or liquidise the soup for about 1 minute.

■ To serve cold, chill and scatter with chopped herbs just before serving. If presenting hot, bring the smooth soup to boiling point, beat the egg yolks with the cream and stir in thoroughly. Reheat but do not allow it to come to the boil.

6 SERVINGS	
kcals	110
kJ	460
CHO	5 g
Fibre	0

VARIATION

Curried Cucumber Soup

ADD 10 ml (2 tsp) curry powder with the flour. Serve hot or cold.

QUICK MEALS

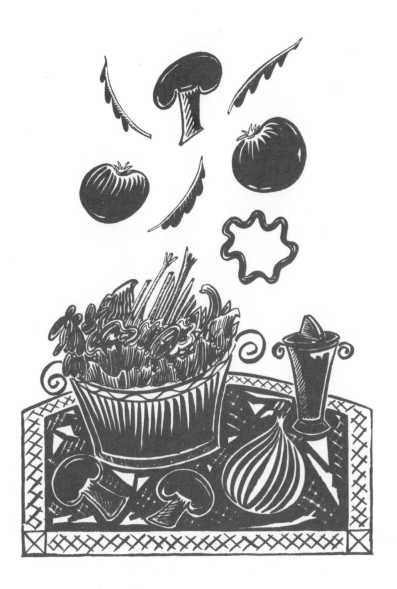

IT IS VERY IMPORTANT for diabetics to be able to prepare and cook a meal quickly, for few things can upset their balance more than irregular meal times. Therefore, it is wise to make sure that foods such as eggs, cheese and some form of fat or oil are always in the house. Also, perhaps more particularly, that there is wholemeal bread, rice, pasta or potato available. Other staples are of course dry goods like flour, either wholemeal or white, and a few basic cans of foods as well as seasonings. With these in stock, it is easy to prepare quite a good meal speedily.

I have also given a few recipes for using leftovers as these can often fill the gap quickly. Therefore when cooking rice, pasta, dried beans, or even potatoes, if you live a fairly chaotic life with varying hours, then it is wise to cook more than you want for one meal as it can be combined with other foods for another meal.

BONED CHICKEN BREASTS

BONED CHICKEN BREASTS are one of the most useful food items for a good quick meal. They come in different sizes with the weight and price marked.

Their uses are myriad; ranging from simply turning them in a little egg and breadcrumbs and frying in a very little oil, to stuffing them and then either baking or poaching.

You should skin them before use, though many chicken breasts are already skinned when bought. Turn them inner side up and you will see, about half-way across, is a flap, like a small pocket. With a sharp knife, you can enlarge this a little, but do not cut right through. Into this 'pocket', you can put a variety of stuffings. Here are some I am fond of, which are not too fattening:

1) Curd or cottage cheese mashed with finely chopped herbs and seasoning.

2) Curd or cottage cheese mashed with a scattering of freshly grated Parmesan cheese, a pinch of freshly grated nutmeg and seasoning.

3) A thin slice of a good cooking cheese, such as Gruyère, Cheddar or Cheshire, with a thin piece of ham, cut to the same size, on top. A smear of mustard can be added, if liked.

4) Chopped mushrooms mixed with chopped, grilled crispy bacon.

5) Wholemeal breadcrumbs, finely chopped herbs and a little grated onion.

6) Cooked apple mixed with cooked, chopped ham or cooked bacon and a pinch of dried sage. The best way of cooking is to poach the breasts in a little dry cider or chicken stock, thickened a little with 10 ml (2 tsp) arrowroot.

7) Dried apricots, soaked, chopped and mixed with some chopped walnuts.

The possibilities are endless and you will enjoy thinking up some of your own. After stuffing, the 'pocket' should be secured with a wooden cocktail stick before cooking.

Fruit Stuffed Chicken Breasts

FOR THIS DISH, you can use either fresh or canned apricots or peaches. If using canned, be sure they are in their natural juice, not sugar syrup.

INGREDIENTS
450 g (1 lb) ripe apricots, peaches or nectarines
2 medium boned chicken breasts
sea salt
little paprika
small pinch of ground cinnamon
5–10 ml (1–2 tsp) sunflower oil
1 small onion, skinned and finely chopped
300 ml ($\frac{1}{2}$ pint) chicken stock, dry cider or dry white wine
150 ml ($\frac{1}{4}$ pint) juice from the fresh fruit after cooking (or can juices)
15 ml (1 tbsp) arrowroot
5 ml (1 tsp) chopped fresh tarragon or 1.25 ml ($\frac{1}{4}$ tsp) dried
freshly ground black pepper
SERVES 2

■ If the fruit is fresh, skin and stone it. Slice all the fruit. Turn the chicken breasts inside uppermost and enlarge the pockets slightly. Stuff them with some of the sliced fruit and secure with wooden cocktail sticks. Season the breasts all over with the salt, paprika and cinnamon.

■ Put the remaining sliced fruit into a saucepan and barely cover with water. Bring to the boil, then simmer until just cooked but not mushy. Cool, drain and reserve the juice.

■ If using canned fruit, no skinning or stoning is needed, simply drain, reserving the can juices, then proceed as above. Again, put the remaining fruit into a saucepan with the can juices, bring to the boil but do not simmer for more than 1 minute. Cool, drain and reserve the juice.

■ Heat the oil, preferably in a non-stick pan, and cook the chicken breasts on both sides for 2–3 minutes. Lift them carefully out on to a shallow, ovenproof dish. Put the onion in the pan and cook very gently until soft and golden. Add the remaining fruit, the stock and the fruit juice, just under 150 ml ($\frac{1}{4}$ pint). Stir well and simmer for 2–3 minutes.

■ Blend the arrowroot with the remaining fruit juice until quite smooth, then quickly add to the hot liquid in the pan, stirring all the time. When it has thickened, season and pour over the chicken.

■ Scatter the tarragon and black pepper over the chicken breasts. Cook at 190°C (375°F) mark 5 for about 30–40 minutes or until the chicken is tender. If liked, serve with fresh runner beans and boiled brown rice, or well puréed potatoes.

2 SERVINGS	
kcals	490
kJ	2050
CHO	20 g
Fibre	5 g

Corn, Ham and Mushroom Casserole

THIS IS AN EXCELLENT DISH for using up leftovers of ham, chicken or turkey. I find it particularly handy after Christmas. Mixtures of these meats can also be used, in fact, whatever you have available. If you prefer, it can all be vegetarian, using more cheese and vegetables.

INGREDIENTS
225 g (8 oz) sweetcorn kernels, cooked, frozen or canned, drained
15 ml (1 tbsp) oil, butter or margarine
1 medium onion, skinned and finely sliced
1 garlic clove, skinned and crushed
2–3 medium tomatoes, skinned and chopped, or canned, drained
100 g (4 oz) mushrooms, chopped
salt and freshly ground black pepper
75 g (3 oz) Cheddar cheese, grated
up to 275 g (10 oz) cooked ham, turkey or chicken, or a mixture, cubed
2.5 ml ($\frac{1}{2}$ tsp) dried tarragon
SERVES 4

■ If using fresh corn, cook in boiling salted water until tender; removing from the cob if whole. Drain, cool and reserve. If using canned corn, make sure that it is whole kernel and without sugar added; drain and reserve.

■ Heat the oil in a pan and lightly fry the onion, then add the garlic and cook until soft. Put in the tomatoes, stir and allow to soften. Add the mushrooms and, with a slice, turn the mixture and season well. Add a little of the juice, if using canned tomatoes, but do not over-moisten the dish.

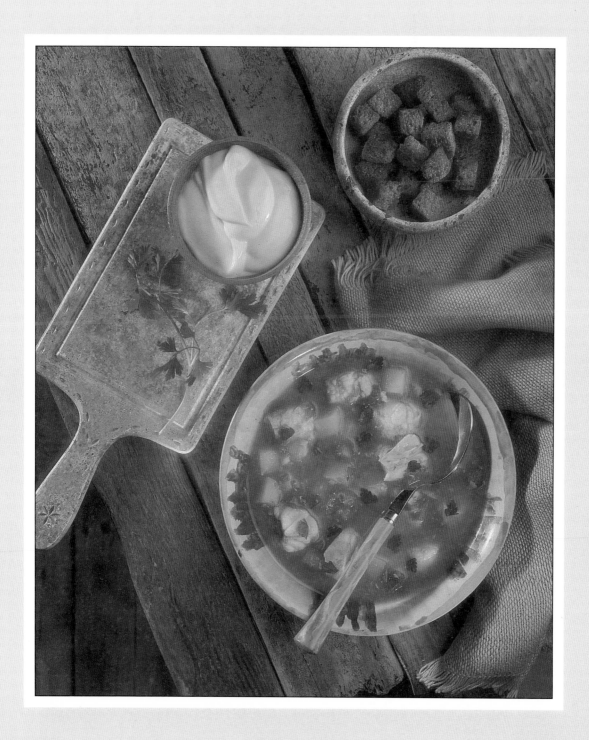

Fish Soup (page 22)

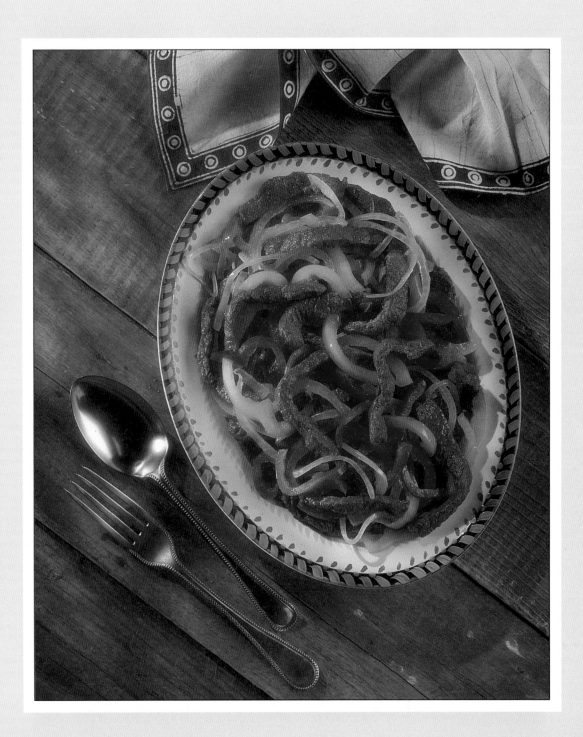

Beef with Peppers (page 70)

■ Put a thin layer of the vegetable mixture in an ovenproof casserole and cover with a sprinkling of the cheese. Add all the meat or poultry, the tarragon and a little seasoning, but do not use too much salt. Add another thin layer of cheese, then cover with the remaining vegetable mixture, smoothing the top and scattering over the remaining cheese evenly.

■ Bake at 190°C (375°F) mark 5 for about 20 minutes or until the cheese is melted and browning.

4 SERVINGS	
kcals	245
kJ	1025
CHO	10 g
Fibre	5 g

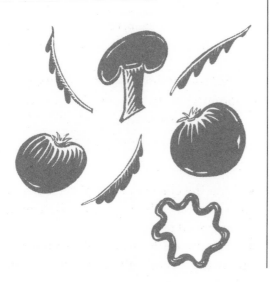

Gratin of Eggs

THIS IS ANOTHER VERY SIMPLE yet satisfying dish. Allow 2 eggs per person.

INGREDIENTS
small knob of butter
6–8 eggs, size 2
90–120 ml (6–8 tbsp) single cream or top of the milk
few drops of Tabasco sauce or Chilli sherry relish (see page 147)
salt and freshly ground black pepper
50–75 g (2–3 oz) hard cheese, grated
SERVES 3 – 4

■ Lightly butter an ovenproof dish all over. Carefully break the eggs into it, making sure that the yolks do not break. Mix the cream with the Tabasco or Chilli sherry relish and season to taste, then spoon it over the eggs. Sprinkle the cheese over the top.

■ Bake at 200°C (400°F) mark 6 for about 12–15 minutes for soft eggs, 20 minutes for medium and 25 minutes if you like them very hard.

3 SERVINGS		4 SERVINGS	
kcals	385	kcals	335
kJ	1610	kJ	1400
CHO	Negligible	CHO	Negligible
Fibre	0	Fibre	0

VARIATIONS

ADD A FEW PIECES of chopped ham or cooked bacon or sautéed mushrooms.

If you have a little cold rice or pasta left over, this can be used as a base to make a more substantial meal.

Mexican Eggs

A VERY PIQUANT DISH which can be made with either raw or hard-boiled eggs.

INGREDIENTS
8 eggs, size 2, raw or hard-boiled (see method)
425 g (15 oz) can tomatoes
175 g (6 oz) can sweetcorn kernels, with no added sugar, drained
½ pepper, cored, deseeded and chopped (optional)
1 medium onion, skinned and finely chopped
1 garlic clove, skinned and crushed
salt and freshly ground black pepper
cayenne pepper
100 g (4 oz) soft cheese, preferably Mozzarella, sliced
SERVES 4

■ For hard-boiled eggs, boil them for 10 minutes. Soak in cold water, then shell.

■ Put the tomatoes and their juice into a bowl. Mix in the corn, pepper if using, onion and garlic, and season to taste with the salt, pepper and cayenne pepper.

■ Put a layer of the tomato and corn mixture on the bottom of an ovenproof dish. If using raw eggs, simply break them in, keeping the yolks whole. If using the hard-boiled eggs, cut them in half lengthwise and arrange them on top of the tomato and corn mixture. Cover with the remainder of the mixture. Lay the cheese over the top.

■ Bake at 200°C (400°F) mark 6 for about 30 minutes or a little longer until the top is golden and bubbling. Serve hot with potato purée or boiled rice.

4 SERVINGS	
kcals	320
kJ	1340
CHO	10 g
Fibre	4 g

VARIATIONS

COVER THE TOP with mashed potato before adding the cheese to make a complete dish.

Leftover pieces of ham or chicken etc. can also be added with the eggs.

Chicken Livers with Bacon and Mushrooms

DELICIOUS ON TOAST, with rice or potatoes and a green vegetable.

INGREDIENTS
450 g (1 lb) chicken livers
seasoned wholemeal flour
15 ml (1 tbsp) sunflower oil
1 medium onion, skinned and finely chopped
4 rashers streaky bacon, derinded and chopped
175 g (6 oz) mushrooms, cut in half if large
150 ml (¼ pint) red wine or chicken stock
pinch of tarragon
salt and freshly ground black pepper
SERVES 4

■ Trim the chicken livers of the sac and any skin or membranes, then roll them in the seasoned flour.

■ Heat the oil in a pan and soften the onion and bacon, lifting out the onion before it colours but letting the bacon become a little crisp before removing. Reduce the heat and soften the mushrooms but do not allow them to crisp. Remove from the pan.

▋ Raise the heat, put in the chicken livers and brown them on the outside all over while remaining just pink within. Add the wine or stock, tarragon and seasoning. Mix well, allow to bubble until the sauce is slightly thickened, but do not boil too rapidly or the livers will toughen.

▋ Return the onion, bacon and mushrooms to the pan, stir once or twice so that all the ingredients are well mixed.

4 SERVINGS	
kcals	345
kJ	1445
CHO	Negligible
Fibre	2 g

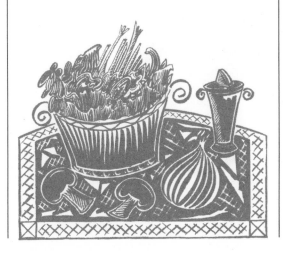

Mushrooms under a Cloche

A FAVOURITE DISH OF MY FATHER'S, this recipe originated in the 18th century. It makes a delicious first course or, if enough mushrooms are used, a light meal. There is, perhaps, no way in which cooked mushrooms have more flavour and the bread, impregnated with the butter and mushroom juices, has a quality which is beyond description! It is easier to serve to a number of people if each serving is baked individually in a small covered dish.

INGREDIENTS
450 g (1 lb) medium mushrooms
225 g (8 oz) butter
5 thick slices of white bread
salt and freshly ground black pepper
SERVES 4

▋ Wipe the mushrooms with a damp cloth and remove the stalks, but do not peel them, leave whole. Lightly butter a large ovenproof dish or individual dishes.

▋ Remove the crusts from the bread slices and cover the bottom of the dish or dishes with a layer of bread. Arrange the mushrooms in a pyramid on the bread, seasoning and liberally buttering each layer. Put a dot of butter on the topmost mushroom. Cover with the lid.

▋ Bake at 220°C (425°F) mark 7 for about 30 minutes.

4 SERVINGS	
kcals	515
kJ	2145
CHO	20 g
Fibre	4 g

Spanish Omelette

NOT ONLY IS THIS OMELETTE very easy to make as it isn't folded over, but it can be eaten hot, or cold on a picnic. It is also a very handy dish for using leftover vegetables and very small pieces of chopped ham, cooked bacon or chicken.

INGREDIENTS

4 eggs, size 5
15 ml (1 tbsp) sunflower oil
1 small to medium onion, skinned and finely chopped
2 tomatoes, skinned and coarsely chopped
½ pepper, cored, deseeded and chopped, or 50 g (2 oz) mushrooms, chopped
2 small cooked potatoes, peeled and thinly sliced
1 garlic clove, skinned and crushed
25–50 g (1–2 oz) cooked ham, bacon or chicken, chopped, or 1–2 slices of skinned salami, chopped
salt and freshly ground black pepper
pinch of dried tarragon
10 ml (2 tsp) chopped fresh parsley or chives

SERVES 2

▌ Beat the eggs in a bowl, add 5 ml (1 tsp) cold water and beat again. Leave for a few minutes, covered, in a cool place.

▌ Heat the oil over a medium heat in a pan and sauté the vegetables in the order given until all are soft but not mushy or coloured. Add the meats last and allow them to heat through. Season to taste.

▌ Season and beat the eggs again. Increase the heat slightly and pour the eggs evenly over the filling, tipping the pan a little if necessary. Lift the omelette with a spatula and, when it is golden underneath, remove the pan from the heat.

▌ Scatter the tarragon over the omelette. Put the omelette under the grill to cook the top, which should still be runny. When the omelette is just set, slip it on to a warmed dish. Alternatively, cut in half in the pan and slip on to 2 warmed serving plates. Sprinkle with parsley. A salad makes a good accompaniment.

2 SERVINGS	
kcals	310
kJ	1295
CHO	15 g
Fibre	3 g

VARIATION

IF LIKED, sprinkle the top with grated Parmesan cheese, or a little grated hard cheese before grilling; this gives a glossy finish and makes the omelette puff up more.

Chilli con Carne

A VERY QUICK, satisfying family meal, particularly appreciated by younger diabetics. Prepared without the beans, this dish will freeze well for 2 months. Add the drained beans when reheating. Serve with crusty bread or boiled rice and a green salad.

INGREDIENTS
15 ml (1 tbsp) oil
1 medium to large onion, skinned and finely chopped
450 g (1 lb) lean minced beef
425 g (15 oz) can tomatoes
15 ml (1 tbsp) tomato purée
2 garlic cloves, skinned and crushed
10 ml (2 tsp) chilli powder or to taste
2.5 ml ($\frac{1}{2}$ tsp) ground cumin
2.5 ml ($\frac{1}{2}$ tsp) ground marjoram or 5 ml (1 tsp) dried
salt and freshly ground black pepper
425 g (15 oz) can kidney beans or use home-cooked (see page 86)
SERVES 4

■ Heat the oil in a pan and lightly fry the onion until soft and golden but not brown. Push to one side and add the beef, breaking it up so that it is level in the pan. Brown quickly, then stir in the onion and allow the meat to become quite well cooked.

■ Drain the tomatoes and reserve the juice. Chop the tomatoes and add to the meat, and then gradually pour in the juice, stirring all the time. When it bubbles, add the tomato purée, garlic, chilli powder, cumin, marjoram and seasoning. Stir well, bring to the boil and simmer for about 15 minutes.

■ Drain the beans and add them to the pan, stirring well. Adjust the seasoning, including the chilli powder. Heat through.

4 SERVINGS	
kcals	295
kJ	1235
CHO	25 g
Fibre	9 g

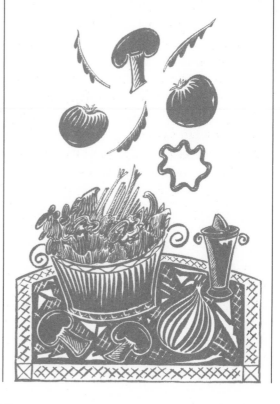

Spinach Baked Omelette

TO MAKE THIS TEMPTING OMELETTE more substantial, serve with a mushroom or parsley sauce.

INGREDIENTS

900 g (2 lb) spinach, washed, drained and coarsely chopped
50 g (2 oz) butter or margarine
6 eggs, size 3
40 g (1½ oz) hard cheese, grated
few drops of Tabasco sauce or Chilli pepper relish (see page 147)
pinch of ground mace
600 ml (1 pint) mushroom or parsley sauce, to serve (optional)

SERVES 4

■ Cook the spinach in a covered saucepan with only 45 ml (3 tbsp) water for 4–5 minutes. Drain and squeeze dry in a chinois sieve or colander. Return the spinach to the saucepan, add the butter and cook over a low heat, turning it over until well coated. Season, but do not add too much salt as there is salt in cheese.

■ Beat the eggs, add 5 ml (1 tsp) water, beat again and add the cheese, Tabasco and mace.

■ Oil a fairly deep 20 cm (8 inch) ovenproof dish and warm it for a few minutes in the oven. Pour in half the beaten egg. Bake at 180°C (350°F) mark 4 for 2 minutes or until the egg is just set.

■ Lay the spinach on top of the set eggs, cover with the remainder of the beaten egg. Bake for 15 minutes or until the top is set and golden. Turn out the omelette on to a warmed dish.

4 SERVINGS	
kcals	325
kJ	1360
CHO	5 g
Fibre	0

VARIATION

COOKED PEAS OR BEANS make a good alternative to spinach.

Lamb and Courgette Kebabs

IT IS POSSIBLE, now, to buy lean cubes of lamb ready for a kebab, or you can cube the meat yourself. Alternatives to lamb are cubes of lamb's liver, kidneys (skinned and halved), bacon or a firm fish such as monkfish. Allow 2 full skewers each.

INGREDIENTS

450 g (1 lb) lean lamb, cubed
450 g (1 lb) courgettes, trimmed
8–10 bay leaves
For the marinade
10 ml (2 tsp) olive oil
1 large garlic clove, skinned and crushed
10 ml (2 tsp) mild curry paste
30 ml (2 tbsp) freshly squeezed lemon juice
sea salt

SERVES 4

■ Mix all the marinade ingredients well together. Put the lamb cubes into a shallow bowl and pour the marinade over them. Turn the lamb cubes in the marinade to ensure that they are individually coated. Set aside, covered, in a cool place for 1 hour.

■ Cut the courgettes into rounds about 0.5 cm (¼ inch) thick. If any of the bay leaves are extra large, break them in two. Take a skewer and make up the kebab, starting with a half bay leaf, a cube of lamb, then a courgette round, then a half bay leaf and so on until the skewer is full.

■ When all the kebabs are made, heat the grill, line the grill pan with foil dull side up, and lay the kebabs on the foil. Put the kebabs under the grill and cook, turning them periodically, until all sides are cooked but not too browned.

4 SERVINGS	
kcals	230
kJ	955
CHO	5 g
Fibre	0

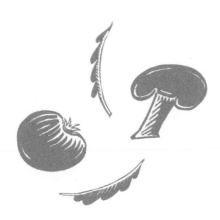

Pipérade Basquaise

A BASQUE DISH WHICH I have often found useful as a supper dish for unexpected guests. If serving with boiled rice, brown rice gives the best flavour. Put a portion of rice on each plate and put the pipérade on top.

INGREDIENTS
30 ml (2 tbsp) oil
1 large onion, skinned and finely chopped
3 garlic cloves, skinned and finely chopped or crushed
2 large red peppers, cored, deseeded and finely sliced, or 1 small can of pimientos, drained
700 g (1½ lb) tomatoes, skinned and chopped, or canned, drained
2.5 ml (½ tsp) dried marjoram
salt and freshly ground black pepper
6 medium sausages or rashers bacon
6 eggs, size 2, or 8 eggs, size 3
SERVES 4

■ Heat the oil in a pan and soften the onion and garlic, but do not allow them to colour. Add the peppers, tomatoes, marjoram and seasoning and sweat gently over a moderate heat. As the juices run out, raise the heat a little to get rid of the excess moisture, but do not let the mixture overcook as it should remain fresh tasting.

■ Meanwhile, grill the sausages or bacon. Chop them and keep warm.

■ Add the unbeaten eggs to the tomato mixture and stir quickly, allowing the eggs to scramble creamily around the vegetables. Turn on to a warmed dish and serve with the sausages or bacon around.

4 SERVINGS	
kcals	505
kJ	2105
CHO	20 g
Fibre	4 g

SOUFFLÉS

SOUFFLÉS ARE ONE OF the most impressive dishes for a quick meal, but the idea of making them appears to frighten most non-professional cooks. Let me reassure you, if you can separate and beat eggs, and make a passable white sauce, then you are a good way there! One other thing; soufflés share one very important point with women—**they should never be kept waiting**! Guests must wait for the soufflé, just as they would in a restaurant. A large soufflé takes about 35 minutes to bake. Small individual cocotte pots filled with a soufflé mixture take only 15–20 minutes to bake and make an excellent first course.

Small amounts of leftover food become transformed. Some suggested fillings are spinach, cauliflower, cheese, smoked fish, shellfish, chicken, ham or tongue. A very little of these is enough to give character to the dish. Always add an extra egg white to a soufflé mixture which has a fairly dense filling such as puréed vegetables, fish, poultry or shellfish.

An electric beater is not the best utensil for producing whisked egg whites for soufflés. A rotary hand beater is better, but best of all is a wire whisk or flat wire whip. Do not whisk the egg whites for soufflés in a plastic bowl or in one which may have the merest trace of fat, grease or oil. Use a wooden spoon for mixing the ingredients together subsequently.

Here are some time and temper savers:

1) The basic roux, before the eggs are added, can be made ahead of time and stored in the refrigerator, covered, for several hours. Take it out an hour before using. Small individual soufflés can be completely prepared, poured into their dishes and refrigerated likewise, but should also be allowed to reach room temperature before baking.

2) A well known chef's trick I sometimes employ: sprinkle a pinch of corn-flour on to the egg whites as they are being whisked. This helps the soufflé to hold up longer.

3) If the basic roux is made with corn-flour instead of flour, the soufflé can be reheated with some success, but it doesn't rise quite so dramatically. Stand the cooked soufflé in a bain-marie or pan of hot water and reheat for 15 minutes at 190°C (375°F) mark 5.

4) A 3 egg soufflé needs a 1.1 litre (2 pint) dish; serves 2–3.

A 4–5 egg soufflé needs a 1.7 litre (3 pint) dish; serves 4–5.

A 6–8 egg soufflé needs a 2.3 litre (4 pint) dish; serves 6–8.

Cheese Soufflé

THE SIMPLEST SOUFFLÉ OF ALL to make; the ingredients are usually in every kitchen.

INGREDIENTS
40 g (1½ oz) butter or margarine
40 g (1½ oz) plain flour
300 ml (½ pint) skimmed milk
salt and cayenne pepper
pinch of dry English mustard powder (not whole-grain)
175 g (6 oz) Cheddar cheese, grated
4 egg yolks, size 2, beaten
4 egg whites, size 2
few drops of Chilli sherry relish (see page 147) or Tabasco sauce (optional)
SERVES 4

▪ Have ready a 1.7 litre (3 pint) soufflé dish or deep china or earthenware casserole. It is best to avoid metal and it is most important that it is **ungreased**.

▪ Melt the butter in a medium saucepan over a low heat, without letting it colour, blend in the flour and cook for 1 minute. Take off the heat and gradually stir in the milk to make a smooth mixture. Put back on a medium heat, stirring all the time until the sauce is smooth and thick. Add the seasonings, then the grated cheese, stirring until it melts and blends in. Remove from the heat, stirring briskly.

▪ While off the heat, gradually add the beaten egg yolks, mixing well. Whisk the egg whites until stiff but not dry. With a metal spoon, gently fold in the egg whites, a little to begin with, then the remainder, making sure that they are evenly mixed in.

▪ Pour the mixture into the dish or dishes and smooth the top. If a 'top hat' effect is liked, trace a circle on the top, about 2.5 cm (1 inch) from the edge of the dish, this allows the soufflé to rise higher in the middle.

▪ Bake at 200°C (400°F) mark 6 for about 20–25 minutes, depending on the exact performance of your oven, baking on a centre shelf.

NOTE: The oven temperature given above is for a French style soufflé, which has a crisp, brown outside and a soft centre. If a drier soufflé is preferred, bake at 180°C (350°F) mark 4 for 50 minutes on the centre shelf. The middle of the soufflé will then be firm but the texture will be less creamy. The soufflé will not rise as high, though it will hold up longer.

4 SERVINGS	
kcals	405
kJ	1695
CHO	10 g
Fibre	0

VARIATIONS

Spinach Soufflé

THE INGREDIENTS ARE SIMILAR to the last recipe, except that 1 egg white, size 2, and 225 g (8 oz) well squeezed puréed cooked spinach are added, together with a generous 15 ml (1 tbsp) grated Parmesan cheese and a good pinch of freshly grated nutmeg.

These amounts also work well for flaked, cooked, smoked fish, puréed cooked crab, puréed cooked cauliflower and so on.

For a smaller soufflé, the amounts of all ingredients can be halved.

Leftover Dishes

I OFTEN COOK MORE PASTA, rice or dried beans than will be used at one meal, as these can form the basis for quick meals another time. Do not discard leftover vegetables, for these too can be used in soups and other dishes. Here are some of my favourites.

Pasta

IF YOU HAVE very little pasta left, then it can be added to vegetable soup, making a kind of minestrone; the same applies to cooked beans.

It can be very good as a salad with some thinly sliced raw peppers, onions and radishes, then dressed with freshly squeezed lemon juice and natural yogurt. Leftover pasta will not dry up if thinly coated in a little oil.

For larger leftovers, the following dishes are quick to make.

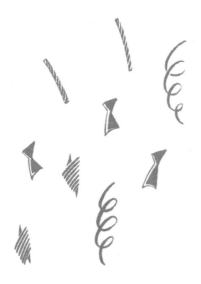

Pasticcio

PASTICCIO IS A POPULAR DISH in my house. You can use either all meat, all vegetables or a mixture of both for this adaptable dish.

INGREDIENTS
30 ml (2 tbsp) sunflower oil
2 medium onions, skinned and thinly sliced
450 g (1 lb) lean minced beef
425 g (15 oz) can of tomatoes
salt and freshly ground black pepper
2.5 ml ($\frac{1}{2}$ tsp) ground cinnamon
1.25 ml ($\frac{1}{4}$ tsp) grated nutmeg
225 g (8 oz) short cut macaroni or pasta shapes, cooked and cold
50 g (2 oz) Parmesan cheese, grated
3 eggs, size 4
150 ml ($\frac{1}{4}$ pint) milk
SERVES 6

▮ Heat the oil in a pan and sauté the onions until just golden. Pour off any excess oil and add the meat, breaking it up well in the pan. Raise the heat a little and brown the meat well. Add the tomatoes, with a little of the juice, mixing them well in, then add the seasoning and spices. Simmer gently until the liquid evaporates. If it becomes too dry before the meat is cooked, add a little more of the tomato juice, just enough to ensure that the mixture is dry just as the meat is finished. Take off the heat.

▮ Lightly oil an ovenproof dish and layer the cooked pasta with the meat mixture, scattering each layer with a little Parmesan cheese, reserving about half of it. Finish with a top layer of pasta. Beat the eggs with the milk and pour over the top.

Scatter on the remaining grated Parmesan.

■ Bake at 180°C (350°F) mark 4 for about 30–40 minutes until the top is puffed up, golden and crisp at the edges.

NOTE: This dish can be prepared ahead of time up to the point where the beaten eggs and milk are poured over the top.

6 SERVINGS	
kcals	360
kJ	1505
CHO	30 g
Fibre	3 g

VARIATION

USE LEFTOVER RICE instead of pasta.

Pasta and Tuna Salad

CANNED, drained tuna and pasta make a pleasant summer lunch; or sardines, drained of oil, can also be used, with some sliced onion, lemon juice and salt. Rice can be used, in place of pasta, in any of the salad dishes.

Cooked Rice

COOKED COLD RICE is best for making fried rice dishes as it has much less of a tendency to 'clump' together when reheated.

Cooked Rice Pilaff

SLICED GREEN BEANS make a pleasant accompaniment to this dish as does a discreet sprinkling of a good soy sauce.

INGREDIENTS
15 ml (1 tbsp) sunflower oil
1 medium onion, skinned and finely chopped
1 red pepper, cored, deseeded and finely chopped
100 g (4 oz) mushrooms, sliced
4 tomatoes, skinned and chopped, or canned, drained
175 g (6 oz) cooked chicken, turkey, ham or pork leftovers
175 g (6 oz) cooked brown or white rice
salt and freshly ground black pepper
chopped fresh parsley, to garnish
SERVES 4

■ Heat the oil in a large pan and lightly sauté the onion and pepper until soft but not coloured. Add the mushrooms and just allow them to soften.

■ Add all the other ingredients, mixing well. Season to taste and, if the contents of the pan appear too dry, add a very little of the tomato juice, but do not over moisten the dish. Garnish with parsley.

NOTE: When using raw rice, allow generous 30 ml (2 tbsp) equalling 75 g (3 oz) for 2 portions. Generous 15 ml (1 tbsp) cooked rice is 30 g (10 g CHO).

4 SERVINGS	
kcals	180
kJ	765
CHO	20 g
Fibre	2 g

Kedgeree

ANOTHER GOOD DISH using leftover boiled rice.

INGREDIENTS
100 g (4 oz) cooked brown or white rice
225 g (8 oz) smoked fish, cooked and flaked
2 eggs, size 2, hard-boiled and quartered
salt and freshly ground black pepper
pinch of freshly grated nutmeg
25 g (1 oz) butter or soft margarine
15 ml (1 tbsp) finely chopped fresh parsley, to garnish
1 lime or lemon, cut into wedges, to serve
SERVES 2

▌ Combine the rice, smoked fish, eggs, seasoning and nutmeg. Put into a lightly greased ovenproof dish and dot the top with the butter.

▌ Bake at 190°C (375°F) mark 5 for 20–30 minutes. Garnish with parsley and serve with lime or lemon wedges.

2 SERVINGS		
kcals	355	
kJ	1490	
CHO	15 g	
Fibre	1 g	(brown rice)
	0 g	(white rice)

Leftover Cooked Beans

WHEN COOKED, any of the dried bean family are most useful for rapid meals. They combine well with brown rice, sliced tomato, garlic, salami and other continental type sausages, making original salads when dressed with olive oil and wine vinegar or with natural Yogurt dressing (see page 114).

Broad Beans

COOKED, cold beans make a most delicious salad with a little sliced onion, a pinch of summer savory or marjoram, seasoned and dressed with olive oil and wine vinegar. Cooked, with a little diced cooked ham and a lot of finely chopped parsley and mixed into a hot pasta, they form a sustaining dish.

See also Omelette Arnold Bennett on page 50 and the Pasta, Rice and Pulses chapter on page 84.

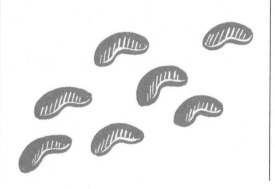

FISH

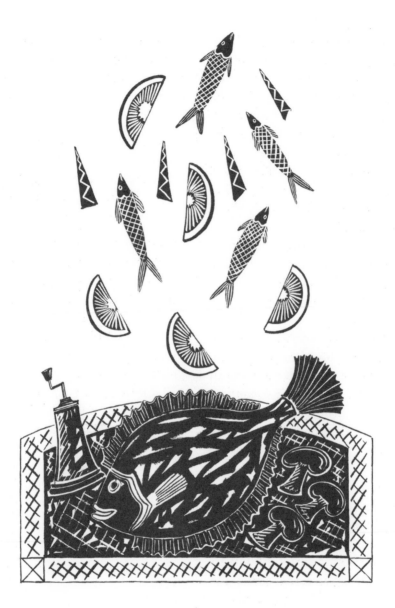

FISH COULD REALLY BE INCLUDED in quick meals, for almost no fish, except large ones such as salmon, take longer than about 30 minutes to cook. They are already prepared for cooking by the fishmonger (and I do recommend buying from one rather than, frozen, from a supermarket, for he will gut and fillet them as well as remove the heads and skin). Bring the bones and skins home with you if you want to make a good fish stock. When strained and cool, fish stock will freeze for a limited time, and be to hand when needed. Indeed, I think of fish as the near perfect convenience food.

Those of you with a microwave oven will know that fish is one of the foods that it cooks best. The fish doesn't shrink and retains that curdy freshness; also, there is no smell. Baking takes away most of the smells but, if cooking on top of the stove, a lidded pan will minimise them.

For diabetics, fish is excellent food as it has, generally speaking, a low fat content, with the exception of herrings, mackerel and salmon. The oils in these oily fish, however, are a good source of vitamins A and D, in which low-fat diets can be deficient. So, if you want to lose weight, or stay slim, always a good idea for a diabetic, eat plenty of white fish. Either grilled, baked or steamed, it is only about 23 calories per 25 g (1 oz).

Don't despise the cheaper fish, such as coley, ling or whiting. Although they are not as full of flavour as some others, they are very good for fish soups, pilaffs and curries.

Another don't, concerns the buying of fish. Personally, I think the very small fillets of lemon sole or plaice a waste of money: it is better to settle for something else. However, if nothing else is available, then be selfish and demand all those without black skin on one side, for, if the tough black skin is left on the plate, I doubt that there is a spoonful of fish to be had! The slightly larger fillets, 18–20 cm (7–8 inches) I stuff, making an excellent, grilled fish 'sandwich', see page 49. You will get much better value by buying a whole, quite large, plaice, then grilling or baking it on the bone. This applies also to bass, John Dory, sea bream and, of course, to small salmon or salmon trout. Not only is the flavour much better this way, but the fish is much cheaper per kg (lb) than fish fillets, steaks or cutlets.

Never buy fish dripping in water, for the water from the melted ice has carried away most of the flavour. If the fish is whole, check that the eyes look bright, shining and fresh, not flattened, sunken and dry.

Always remember, when buying shell-fish, to choose the heaviest, not necessarily the largest; the heaviest will contain the most meat.

Baking Fish

THIS COOKING METHOD is extremely good for diabetics as it not only preserves the flavour but needs no addition of fat; the calorific content is thus kept low. Fish can be baked either with liquids or vegetables, or simply put the cleaned fish on to a piece of slightly oiled foil or grease-proof paper, sprinkle with chopped herbs and a little freshly squeezed lemon juice and wrap securely. Put the parcel on a dish or tray and bake at 190°C (375°F) mark 5 for about 25 minutes per 0.5 kg (1 lb) fish, depending on the kind of fish and the thickness.

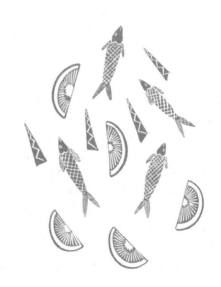

Court Bouillon or Fish Stock

DIETARY FIGURES for this recipe are not given because the solids are removed, making it impossible to determine what nutrients are left in the stock. However, since it is largely made up of water, this should not be a problem!

INGREDIENTS

900 ml (1½ pints) water
150 ml (¼ pint) dry white wine or dry cider
30 ml (2 tbsp) white wine vinegar
450 g (1 lb) white fish heads and trimmings
1 medium onion, skinned and sliced
1 garlic clove, skinned and chopped
1 medium carrot, scraped and sliced
1 celery stalk, trimmed and sliced
1 clove
6 black peppercorns, crushed
1 small bay leaf
1 bouquet garni
salt

MAKES 1 litre (1¾ pints)

▌ Bring the water, wine and vinegar to the boil in a saucepan. Add the fish heads and trimmings, the vegetables and the spices, herbs and seasoning. Cook gently for 1 hour.

▌ Strain and the court bouillon is ready for use. When cool, it may be kept in a screw-topped jar in the refrigerator for about 10 days.

Creamed Cod with Egg and Sultana Sauce

THIS TEMPTING DISH is also good when made with haddock or hake.

INGREDIENTS

700 g (1½ lb) cod fillets
300 ml (½ pint) court bouillon (left)
15 g (½ oz) butter or margarine
15 ml (1 tbsp) flour
300 ml (½ pint) milk, hot
1 hard-boiled egg, size 2, chopped
25 g (1 oz) sultanas or grapes
15 ml (1 tbsp) dry sherry
salt and freshly ground black pepper

SERVES 4

▌ Cook the cod fillets gently in the court bouillon for 20 minutes. Drain and flake the fish into an ovenproof dish.

▌ Melt the butter in a saucepan and blend in the flour evenly. Gradually add the hot milk, stirring constantly. Add the hard-boiled egg, sultanas and sherry and season to taste. Simmer for 3 minutes.

▌ Pour the sauce over the fish. Bake at 180°C (350°F) mark 4 for 20 minutes.

4 SERVINGS	
kcals	255
kJ	1065
CHO	10 g
Fibre	0

Greek Fish Casserole

ANY WHITE FISH or shellfish or a mixture of both can be used.

INGREDIENTS
1.1 kg (2½ lb) fish, skinned and filleted
seasoned flour
15 ml (1 tbsp) oil
1 leek or 1 medium onion, skinned and chopped
450 g (1 lb) ripe tomatoes, skinned and chopped
185 g (6½ oz) can of sweet red peppers, drained and chopped
45–60 ml (3–4 tbsp) white wine
1 large fresh basil leaf or pinch of dried
2 eggs, size 3
150 ml (¼ pint) natural yogurt
50 g (2 oz) cheese, grated
SERVES 6

▐ Cut the fish into small pieces, then roll in the seasoned flour. Heat the oil in a pan and quickly fry the fish until cooked. Remove from the pan. Add the leek and soften, but do not allow to colour. Stir in the tomatoes and peppers and cook for 1 minute. Add the wine and basil and cook until a purée is formed. Season.

▐ Line the bottom of an ovenproof dish with the purée and place the fish pieces on top. Beat the eggs and yogurt together and pour over the fish. Sprinkle with the cheese. Bake at 180°C (350°F) mark 4 for 20–30 minutes or until the top has set.

6 SERVINGS	
kcals	255
kJ	1065
CHO	5 g
Fibre	2 g

Cod à la Bretonne

THIS EASY RECIPE also works well for other white fish, such as hake and whiting.

INGREDIENTS
4 cod fillets
seasoned flour
salt and freshly ground black pepper
2 shallots or 1 small onion, skinned and sliced
225 g (8 oz) mushrooms, sliced
15 ml (1 tbsp) chopped fresh parsley
200 g (7 oz) can tomatoes
150 ml (¼ pint) dry cider or fish stock
25 g (1 oz) cheese, grated
SERVES 4

▐ Roll the fish fillets in the seasoned flour. Lightly grease an ovenproof dish and put in the fish fillets. Season and cover with the shallot or onion, mushrooms and parsley, then the tomatoes and their juice. Season again to taste and pour the cider gently over.

▐ Bake at 180°C (350°F) mark 4 for 20 minutes. Sprinkle the cheese over the top and bake for a further 10 minutes or until the top is golden.

4 SERVINGS	
kcals	215
kJ	900
CHO	5 g
Fibre	2 g

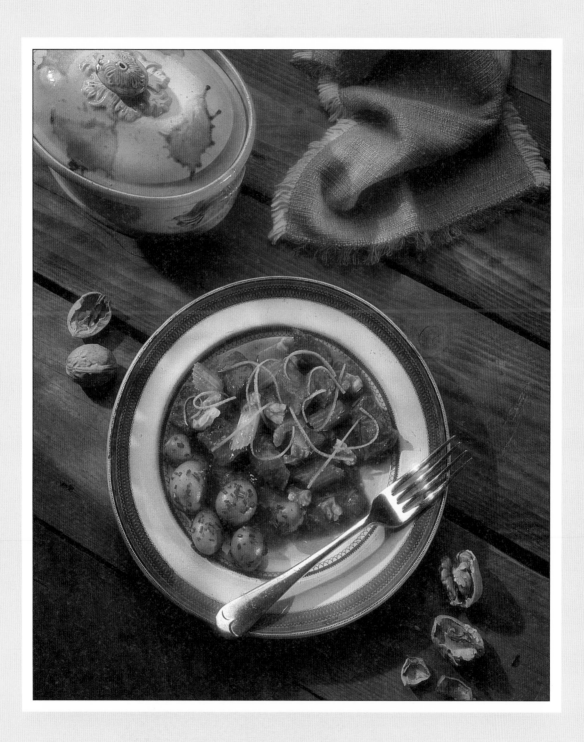

Beef Casserole with Celery and Walnuts (page 69)

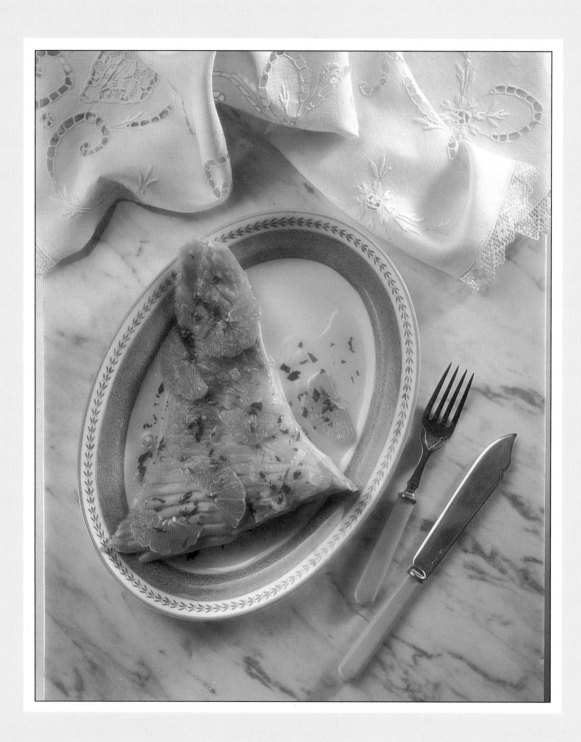

Skate with Orange (opposite)

Lemon Sole Grilled with Cottage Cheese

GRILLING WITH COTTAGE OR CURD CHEESE is an excellent way to cook small fillets. The fish should be filleted right across, so that two whole fillets, the shape of the fish, are obtained from each; your fish-monger will do this for you.

INGREDIENTS

8 lemon sole (whole side) fillets	
15 g ($\frac{1}{2}$ oz) butter or margarine	
15 ml (1 tbsp) finely chopped fresh parsley	
50 g (2 oz) sieved cottage or curd cheese	
salt and freshly ground black pepper	
juice of 1 lemon	
10 ml (2 tsp) oil	

SERVES 4

■ Line the grill pan with oiled foil, dull side up. Lay 4 of the fillets on the foil, skin side down. Lightly butter each.

■ Mix the parsley well into the cheese, season lightly and add the lemon juice. Divide the cheese mixture between the 4 fillets, mounding it a little towards the centre of each. Place the remaining fillets over their matched pairs, so that the skin side is on top. Pour over a dribble of oil.

■ Put the fish under a fairly hot grill to cook until the skin blisters slightly, then carefully turn each pair over and grill the other side. Serve on warmed plates.

4 SERVINGS	
kcals	325
kJ	1360
CHO	0
Fibre	0

Skate with Orange

THE TRIANGULAR, ribbed wings of this fish are sold whole or in portions.

INGREDIENTS

450–700 g (1–1$\frac{1}{2}$ lb) skate wings	
salt and freshly ground black pepper	
25 g (1 oz) butter or margarine	
1 small onion, skinned and finely chopped	
2 small oranges, thin skinned if possible	
5 ml (1 tsp) finely chopped fresh parsley	
5 ml (1 tsp) finely chopped fresh lemon thyme	
squeeze of fresh lemon juice	

SERVES 4

■ Poach the skate wings in a little salted water for about 15–20 minutes. Drain very well, put on to a warmed dish and keep hot.

■ Melt 15 g ($\frac{1}{2}$ oz) of the butter in a pan, add the onion and soften without letting it brown. Peel 1 orange, slice it into rounds and cut each round in half. Add the rest of the butter to the pan and quickly fry the orange slices without browning.

■ Add the juice from the other orange, the herbs, seasoning and a good squeeze of lemon juice. Bring to the boil, pour over the fish and serve.

4 SERVINGS	
kcals	225
kJ	940
CHO	5 g
Fibre	1 g

Grilled John Dory with Fennel

A MOST DELICIOUS SUMMER DISH which requires fresh fennel stalks or fronds.

INGREDIENTS
15 ml (1 tbsp) olive oil
4 thick fennel stalks
900 g (2 lb) whole John Dory, cleaned
salt and freshly ground black pepper
several fennel fronds
1 lemon, cut in wedges, to garnish
SERVES 2 – 3

■ Rub a little olive oil on the base of an oval, flameproof dish which will just fit the fish. Lay the fennel stalks in the dish and put the fish on top. Season. Stuff the gullet of the fish with the fennel fronds. Slash the fish twice diagonally and pour over the rest of the olive oil.

■ Preheat the grill and remove the rack from the grill pan. Put the dish into the grill pan. Place under the grill, but not too close, so that the fish will cook without burning, although a few blisters on the skin will merely add to its attractiveness. To test if the fish is cooked through, check that the flesh comes away from the backbone at the thickest part. Serve with the lemon wedges and the remaining fennel fronds as garnish.

2 SERVINGS		3 SERVINGS	
kcals	470	kcals	310
kJ	1960	kJ	1305
CHO	Negligible	CHO	Negligible
Fibre	Negligible	Fibre	Negligible

Omelette Arnold Bennett

A GREAT FAVOURITE OF MINE, this omelette is excellent followed by a crisp salad.

INGREDIENTS
175 g (6 oz) smoked haddock, cooked, flaked
15 g (½ oz) hard cheese, grated
15 g (½ oz) butter or margarine
6 eggs, size 3, beaten
30 ml (2 tbsp) double cream
SERVES 2

■ Mix the flaked fish with the cheese and pepper to taste. Heat the butter in a heavy pan until it foams. Pour in the beaten eggs before the butter browns. Mix with a spatula, so that they form a mound in the middle, then tip the pan around so that none of the pan base is left uncovered.

■ While some of the egg is still liquid, add the fish and cheese mixture evenly all over. After 1 minute, take from the heat and pour over the cream.

■ Put under a hot grill for 2–3 minutes until the top becomes golden and bubbling. Serve, without folding, on a warmed dish or 2 warmed plates.

2 SERVINGS	
kcals	470
kJ	1960
CHO	0
Fibre	0

Plaice Lahori

YOU MUST HAVE A LARGE PLAICE for this dish, not those wafer-thin little fillets one sometimes sees. When properly carried out, this recipe will make even dogfish or monkfish delicious, but the cooking time needs to be increased.

INGREDIENTS
4 large plaice fillets
15 ml (1 tbsp) oil, melted butter or margarine
For the marinade
2 medium onions, skinned and grated
juice of 1 lemon
10 ml (2 tsp) chopped fresh coriander or 1.25 ml (¼ tsp) dried
1 garlic clove, skinned and crushed
pinch of turmeric
10 ml (2 tsp) chopped fresh root ginger
2 medium to large ripe tomatoes, skinned and pulped
salt and freshly ground black pepper
SERVES 4

■ Mix the marinade ingredients together well in a bowl. If the fish fillets are very thick, score several times with a knife to allow the marinade to penetrate. Place the fillets in a shallow dish, pour the marinade over and allow to marinate for at least 2 hours.

■ Line a grill pan with foil, brush over the surface with the oil and place under the grill to allow it to become really hot, but do not let the oil discolour. Carefully lift the fillets on to the heated foil and cover them with the remaining marinade. Grill under medium heat for about 7 minutes or until the fish is cooked through. Serve with green beans and brown rice.

4 SERVINGS	
kcals	195
kJ	820
CHO	5 g
Fibre	1 g

Soused Herrings

THIS IS A TRADITIONAL West Country dish which is also very good using mackerel, pilchards or sprats.

INGREDIENTS
8 bay leaves
8 fresh herrings, scaled, heads removed, cleaned and boned
15 black peppercorns
300 ml (½ pint) equal parts of white vinegar and cold milkless tea
SERVES 4

■ Place a bay leaf inside each fish. Lay the fish in an ovenproof dish. Sprinkle the peppercorns over and pour over the vinegar and tea mixture to just cover the fish.
■ Cover and bake at 180°C (350°F) mark 4 for 1 hour. Leave until cold in the liquor. Serve cold with a little of the jelly formed by the cooled liquor.

4 SERVINGS	
kcals	785
kJ	3285
CHO	0
Fibre	0

Salmon or Salmon Trout Baked in Foil

TODAY, except in unusually well equipped kitchens, fish kettles are a rarity and, besides, even when very carefully poached, fish loses considerable flavour to the water. I prefer the method of baking the fish, sealed in oiled foil, as the flavour is superior: and turkey size foil is cheap and readily available too.

INGREDIENTS
1.8 kg (4 lb) whole salmon or salmon trout, cleaned
15 ml (1 tbsp) vegetable oil
squeeze of fresh lemon juice
6 fronds of fresh fennel
SERVES 8

■ Cut off the salmon tail, but leave the head on. Wash well, both inside and out, in cold running water to remove any slime. Pat dry with absorbent kitchen paper. Take 2 thicknesses of cooking foil, arranging them over one another so that the dull side is uppermost. Oil this surface all over and any part that will come in contact with the fish.

■ Use the remainder of the oil to oil the outside of the fish and place it on the oiled foil. Squeeze the lemon juice into the gullet and body cavity and fill both with the fennel fronds. Wrap the fish carefully in the foil, folding into a juice-tight parcel.

■ Carefully lift the packaged fish on to a flat baking tray, lying diagonally across it if your oven is small. Bake at 180°C (350°F) mark 4 for about 45 minutes. If it is to be eaten hot, leave in the foil for 10 minutes to 'set' before opening, skinning and serving. If it is to be eaten cold, skin while still warm and keep covered to prevent it from becoming dry. For sauces for salmon, see pages 108–115.

8 SERVINGS	
kcals	425
kJ	1780
CHO	0
Fibre	0

Grilled Salmon Steaks

FRESH SALMON IS PERFECT simply prepared. Grilled and served with herb butter is an ideal choice.

INGREDIENTS
40 g (1½ oz) butter or margarine
15 ml (1 tbsp) finely chopped fresh parsley
juice of ¼ lemon
50 g (2 oz) butter or margarine
4 salmon steaks
25 g (1 oz) seasoned flour
SERVES 4

■ To make herb butter, work the 40 g (1½ oz) butter with the parsley and lemon juice in a bowl. Cover and chill.

■ Remove the rack from the grill pan and cover the inside of the pan with a double thickness of foil, dull side uppermost. Well grease with butter. Heat the grill and put the foil lined grill pan under it but not too close.

■ Dust the salmon steaks lightly with the seasoned flour on both sides. Remove the grill pan from the heat and turn the floured salmon steaks over in the hot butter, so that both sides are coated. Return to the grill and cook for about 8 minutes or until they are done, depending on the thickness, and are just a browny-gold at the edges. If they are thick steaks, they may have to be turned after 5 minutes.

■ Put a quarter of the herb butter on top of each steak and serve on warmed plates.

4 SERVINGS	
kcals	495
kJ	2070
CHO	5 g
Fibre	0

Salmon, Stuffed and Baked

IF LIKED, serve the salmon with Yogurt spiced sauce on page 113.

INGREDIENTS
2.3 kg (5 lb) whole salmon, cleaned
salt
juice of $\frac{1}{2}$ lemon
225 g (8 oz) monkfish, cod or haddock, skinned and filleted
6 fennel fronds or 2.5 ml ($\frac{1}{2}$ tsp) fennel seeds
pinch of dried tarragon
1 egg yolk
15–30 ml (1–2 tbsp) single cream
15 g ($\frac{1}{2}$ oz) butter or margarine
150 ml ($\frac{1}{4}$ pint) dry white wine or dry cider
SERVES 10

■ Cut off the salmon tail. Wash well, both inside and out, gullet included, in cold running water to remove slime. Pat dry with absorbent kitchen paper. Rub the inside of the fish with a little salt and half of the lemon juice. Put aside in a cool place.

■ Lightly poach the monkfish or other fish in water barely to cover and drain. Blend the fish in a food processor or liquidiser with 2 fennel fronds, the tarragon, egg yolk, cream, salt and the remainder of the lemon juice.

■ Fill the interior of the fish with this stuffing and secure the opening with small metal skewers. Place the fish carefully in a large, buttered ovenproof dish, without bending it. Pour the wine around and cover.

■ Bake at 180°C (350°F) mark 4 for about 50 minutes–1 hour. Take out, leave covered for 10 minutes to 'set', skin the upper side and garnish with the remaining fennel.

10 SERVINGS	
kcals	375
kJ	1570
CHO	0
Fibre	0

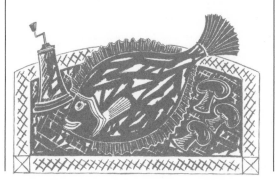

POULTRY AND GAME

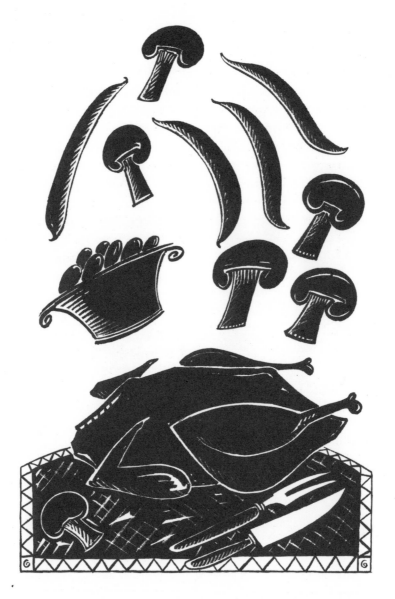

CHICKEN IS LOW IN CALORIES and good value these days, especially if you use the carcass afterwards for making soup. I put my carcasses into the freezer and, when I have two or three, make a good stock with them, adding some herbs and plenty of tarragon, either fresh or dried, and sometimes using a few chicken stock cubes as well. Stock made in this way always jellies when chilled. It is simple to de-fat too if chilled in a tall plastic container, the solidified fat being easy to remove from the top. Leave the fat on though, until just before you are going to use the stock, as it seals it and helps to keep in the flavour. Stock will keep perfectly for 5–6 days in the refrigerator. It is very good served just as it is, in a soft jelly, as a cold soup, and makes a good basis for many other excellent soups, both cold and hot.

An easy gazpacho-type soup can be made in 5 minutes with a liquidiser or food processor by combining the defatted stock with some skinned tomatoes, a little skinned onion and deseeded peppers. It makes a perfect base for a lettuce soup, too.

A boiled chicken is useful for the impromptu picnic as well as for making other more elaborate dishes. Unfortunately, fowl can be overdone, so that the wings and legs fall off and the breast becomes dry when cold. I have a perfect method (see right), taught to me by a Chinese friend, making the boiling easy and reliable, but it must be followed *exactly*.

Autumn is the only time of year when many varieties of game are available, though some are expensive at the beginning of the season. Bringing its own richness not only in food but in the exotic colourings of foliage and berries, autumn is like a glorious last fling on the part of nature, before winter. In the country, it is sometimes easier and cheaper to obtain pheasant than in town. If you do find them reasonably priced, it is wise to buy them for, after being adequately hung, they freeze very well. It is most important to stress that they must be hung before freezing, as no amount of hanging afterwards will do any good; they will only go bad.

If you are a fairly small family, try pheasant for Christmas; to me it is much more enjoyable than turkey and one doesn't have it hanging around for ages afterwards! One good plump pheasant will serve 3 people adequately and there is still the carcass to form the basis of a good game soup.

Chinese Method for Boiling a Chicken

WASH THE CHICKEN, inside and out. Rub over with a cut lemon and put 3–5 metal, preferably silver plated, dessert size forks (depending on the size of the bird) into the body cavity—this helps to conduct the heat. Put the chicken into a large saucepan with a lid, with the rest of the lemon, some fresh or dried tarragon, plenty of parsley and 2 chicken stock cubes. Cover the bird with cold water and season with salt and freshly ground black pepper. Bring to the boil and simmer for exactly 15 minutes, take from the heat and leave to stand, covered, in a cool place until *completely cold*.

If it is left to cool, covered, overnight, in the morning, you will have a perfectly boiled chicken, no matter what the size, with no risk of overcooking. Remember, however, to take out the cutlery when the bird is cold. They will have become a little tarnished, but the cleaning is easy if done at once. This method also makes a particularly well flavoured stock, from which a simple chicken soup can be made when defatted.

You can use the chicken to prepare all kinds of dishes, including curries, which entail a certain amount of additional cooking as well.

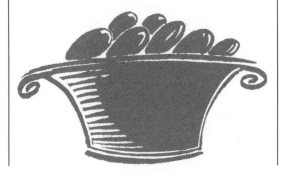

Chicken with Bean Sprouts and Walnuts

A CHINESE-STYLE DISH which is stir-fried, making a speedy main course.

INGREDIENTS

450 g (1 lb) chicken meat, either breast or thigh, boned
15 ml (1 tbsp) soy sauce
15 ml (1 tbsp) dry sherry
1 garlic clove, skinned and crushed
salt
1 egg white
15 ml (1 tbsp) vegetable oil
150 g (5 oz) fresh bean sprouts, or canned, drained
1 medium green pepper, cored, deseeded and cut into strips
50 g (2 oz) walnuts or almonds
For the sauce
45 ml (3 tbsp) chicken stock
5 ml (1 tsp) white wine vinegar
5 ml (1 tsp) soy sauce
5 ml (1 tsp) sesame oil
10 ml (2 tsp) cornflour
SERVES 2 – 3

■ Cut the chicken into small cubes or strips. Mix together the soy sauce, sherry, garlic, salt and egg white in a dish. Add the chicken and marinate for 1 hour.

■ Heat the oil in a pan and fry the chicken for 1 minute, taking care that the pieces are kept separated, then remove and keep hot. Lightly fry the bean sprouts and pepper strips for 3 minutes, stirring well, to soften but do not allow them to colour. Put the chicken back into the pan, add the nuts and stir-fry for 5 minutes.

■ Mix together the sauce ingredients, add them to the pan and stir vigorously until thickened. Serve with boiled brown or white rice.

2 SERVINGS		3 SERVINGS	
kcals	530	kcals	355
kJ	2210	kJ	1475
CHO	10 g	CHO	5 g
Fibre	2 g	Fibre	1 g

VARIATION

PORK STRIPS OR PRAWNS or a mixture of both can be used instead of chicken.

Pollo alla Romana con Peperoni— Roman Chicken

THIS NUTRITIOUS AND DELICIOUS Roman dish can also be made with stewing beef, using 900 g (2 lb) cubed meat, beef stock and increasing the cooking time by 30 minutes.

INGREDIENTS

1.6 kg (3½ lb) roasting chicken, jointed
seasoned flour
30 ml (2 tbsp) oil
450 g (1 lb) mixed red and green peppers, cored, deseeded and cut into strips
pinch of finely chopped fresh rosemary
1 garlic clove, skinned and crushed
150 g (5 oz) canned tomatoes
600 ml (1 pint) chicken stock
salt and freshly ground black pepper
SERVES 4 – 6

Wipe the chicken joints, remove the skin and any fat. Roll them in the seasoned flour. Heat 15 ml (1 tbsp) of the oil in a deep pan and sauté the peppers. Transfer them to a casserole. Add the remaining oil to the pan and sauté the chicken joints until golden all over. Add the rosemary, garlic, tomatoes and stock. Season to taste. Bring to the boil, pour over the peppers in the casserole and mix very well.

Cover and cook at 180°C (350°F) mark 4 for 1½ hours or until tender, checking half way through the cooking time that it is not catching at the bottom and giving the casserole a good stir.

4 SERVINGS		6 SERVINGS	
kcals	355	kcals	235
kJ	1490	kJ	995
CHO	10 g	CHO	5 g
Fibre	2 g	Fibre	1 g

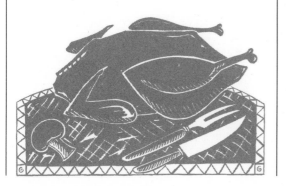

Chicken in Orange Sauce

ADAPTED FOR DIABETICS from a popular Israeli dish, this flavourful dish is easy to prepare.

INGREDIENTS
1.6 kg (3½ lb) chicken, jointed
For the marinade
30 ml (2 tbsp) grated orange rind
450 ml (¾ pint) orange juice
5 ml (1 tsp) fructose
50 g (2 oz) margarine
10 ml (2 tsp) mild mustard
5 ml (1 tsp) salt
thin orange slices, to garnish
SERVES 4 – 6

Lay the chicken joints, skin side downwards, in a greased roasting pan. Mix the ingredients for the marinade well together. Pour over the bird, rub it well in and leave for 1 hour.

Roast at 220°C (425°F) mark 7 for 45 minutes or until tender, basting frequently with the marinade and turning after 30 minutes so that it browns evenly. Put the chicken joints on to a warmed serving dish and keep hot.

Pour the marinade and juices into a saucepan, bring to the boil and simmer until reduced a little. Pour the orange sauce over the chicken, garnish with orange slices and serve.

4 SERVINGS		6 SERVINGS	
kcals	385	kcals	255
kJ	1610	kJ	1070
CHO	10 g	CHO	5 g
Fibre	0	Fibre	0

Chicken Lahori

THIS COLOURFUL DISH FROM INDIA is not hot like a curry, but it is full of flavour. The chicken should marinate for 1 hour at the very least, but the longer you can manage, the better. Overnight in a cool place is not too long if you have a really fresh chicken.

INGREDIENTS
1.6 kg (3½ lb) chicken, cleaned, without giblets
lemon wedges, to serve
For the marinade
1 small onion, skinned and chopped
juice of 1 lemon
10 ml (2 tsp) chopped fresh coriander, or 2.5 ml (½ tsp) ground coriander
1 garlic clove, skinned and chopped
pinch of ground turmeric
10 ml (2 tsp) peeled and chopped fresh root ginger
2 large ripe tomatoes, skinned and chopped, or canned, drained and chopped
salt and freshly ground black pepper
30 ml (2 tbsp) olive oil
SERVES 4 – 6

■ Mix all the marinade ingredients in a deep dish, pounding them well. Add the olive oil and mix together thoroughly. Put the chicken in the dish and rub the marinade in well all over, but especially the breast and legs. Cover and leave in a cool place to marinate for at least 1–2 hours, turning several times. If you have time to marinate it for longer, the flavour will be better.

■ Line a baking tin with foil dull side up, and put the bird in. Pour the marinade over the breast and legs. Wrap the foil loosely around, closing over the top. Roast at 200°C (400°F) mark 6 for 30 minutes, then lower the temperature to 180°C (350°F) mark 4 and continue cooking for 1 hour more.

■ Open out the foil and return to the oven for about 20 minutes so that the top and legs can brown, but make sure that the marinade is not drying up. Put on to a warmed serving dish with the pan juices and serve at once with freshly boiled brown or white rice and lemon wedges.

4 SERVINGS		6 SERVINGS	
kcals	325	kcals	210
kJ	1370	kJ	870
CHO	Negligible	CHO	Negligible
Fibre	Negligible	Fibre	Negligible

VARIATION

THIS DISH CAN ALSO be prepared using a small turkey or with chicken joints. If using chicken joints, when putting them into the foil, make sure to distribute the marinade evenly between them before sealing the foil. Breast or thigh joints are best for this. The cooking time should be about 1½ hours.

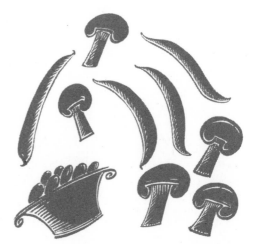

Chicken Korma Curry

THE BOILED CHICKEN, given on page 55, is excellent for this dish. This dish can be cooked the day before and it will only improve in flavour when reheated, but do not scatter the mixture of cardamom and nutmeg over until just before serving.

INGREDIENTS

900 g (2 lb) cooked chicken, without skin, bone or gristle

60 ml (4 tbsp) oil

2 medium onions, skinned and sliced

30 ml (2 tbsp) tomato purée

5 ml (1 tsp) chilli powder or to taste

2 bay leaves

salt

450 ml ($\frac{3}{4}$ pint) chicken stock

5 ml (1 tsp) ground cardamom

5 ml (1 tsp) freshly grated nutmeg

For the marinade

150 ml ($\frac{1}{4}$ pint) natural yogurt

3 garlic cloves, skinned and chopped

10 ml (2 tsp) peeled and chopped fresh root ginger, or 2.5 ml ($\frac{1}{2}$ tsp) ground ginger

5 ml (1 tsp) ground cumin

5 ml (1 tsp) ground coriander

5 ml (1 tsp) ground cloves

5 ml (1 tsp) ground cardamom

5 ml (1 tsp) garam masala

SERVES 4 – 6

▌ Cut the chicken into convenient serving pieces. Mix the yogurt, garlic and marinade spices well together. Rub the chicken with the marinade and leave for 2 hours to marinate, if you have the time to spare, if not leave for 30 minutes.

▌ Meanwhile, heat the oil in a deep pan and soften the onions, but do not let them colour or the result will be bitter. Add the chicken and marinade to the onions, raise the heat and let it bubble up. Add the tomato purée, chilli powder, bay leaves and season to taste with salt. Mix thoroughly, with a wooden spoon, for about 10–15 minutes until the oil separates from the spices.

▌ Add the chicken stock and simmer slowly for about 25 minutes, stirring from time to time. Before serving, mix the ground cardamom and grated nutmeg together and scatter over the top. Serve with boiled brown or white rice.

4 SERVINGS		6 SERVINGS	
kcals	490	kcals	330
kJ	2055	kJ	1370
CHO	10 g	CHO	5 g
Fibre	0	Fibre	0

VARIATION

THIS DISH CAN ALSO be made with 900 g (2 lb) lean, cubed, beef stewing steak. Simmer the steak gently in the marinade for 30 minutes and continue with the recipe but simmer for about 45 minutes after the stock (which should be a beef stock) is added.

Roast Duck Stuffed with Apple and Prunes

FOR BEST RESULTS, rub the duck breast with coarse salt, if possible.

INGREDIENTS
1.8 kg (4 lb) duckling, cleaned
salt and freshly ground black pepper
ground ginger
300 ml ($\frac{1}{2}$ pint) dry cider or dry red wine
3 medium apples, peeled, cored and sliced in rings
15 g ($\frac{1}{2}$ oz) butter or margarine
For the stuffing
30 ml (2 tbsp) oil
1 medium onion, skinned and finely chopped
2 medium cooking apples, peeled, cored and chopped
12 prunes, soaked for 3 hours, stoned and chopped
1.25 ml ($\frac{1}{4}$ tsp) ground sage
1 egg, size 4, beaten
SERVES 3 – 4

■ For the stuffing, heat the oil in a pan and soften the onion, without letting it colour. Add the apples and soften them. Finally add the prunes and sage and season to taste. Take off the heat, put into a small bowl and mix in the egg. Stuff the bird with this mixture and secure the opening.
■ If you have a rack, put this in the roasting pan. Prick the duck all over with a fine pronged fork and rub the breast with the salt, pepper and ginger.

■ Place the duck on the rack and roast at 200°C (400°F) mark 6 towards the top of the oven. Every 20 minutes, remove from the oven and pour off the fat. At the beginning there will not be much but you will be astonished how much fat finally comes out. Be sure to save the fat, which is excellent for many kinds of frying, especially sautéed potatoes, bread etc. This repeated procedure ensures a really crisp, dry skin, so is well worth the trouble.
■ Allow a cooking time of 25–30 minutes per 0.5 kg (1 lb) duck. When the cooking is nearly completed, drain off the fat again, taking care not to pour away the juices beneath the fat. Put the duck on to a warmed serving dish and keep hot.
■ Pour all the remaining pan juices into a medium saucepan and boil on the top of the stove, adding the dry cider or red wine. Bring to the boil, season to taste and keep hot in a sauceboat.
■ Fry the apple rings lightly in the butter, garnish the duck with them and serve accompanied with the cider or wine sauce.

3 SERVINGS		4 SERVINGS	
kcals	290	kcals	220
kJ	1230	kJ	920
CHO	35 g	CHO	25 g
Fibre	10 g	Fibre	7 g

VARIATIONS

DRIED APRICOTS, soaked and chopped, may be used instead of the prunes.

Just before serving, the duck and its garnish can be flamed in a little brandy, heated and ignited in a ladle and poured, flaming, over the bird.

For Apple sauce, see page 107.

Roast Turkey, the French Way

TURKEY IS A DRY BIRD and the difficulty of cooking it with success is that the breast cooks more quickly than the legs, so the breast can get very dry. This is especially likely to happen when the bird is cooked with a fat or oil baste. This French method, using a stock or stock and cider or wine baste, gives a far superior result, keeping the whole bird moist and tender. A variety of stuffings can be used, see pages 116–118: Chestnut stuffing (see page 116) is excellent for the crop.

INGREDIENTS
3.6–4 kg (8–9 lb) turkey, the blue-legged variety is best
10 ml (2 tsp) chopped dried tarragon
25 g (1 oz) butter or margarine
salt and freshly ground black pepper
600 ml (1 pint) giblet stock, chicken stock, dry cider or dry wine

SERVES 8 – 10

■ Make certain that your roasting tin and oven are big enough to take the turkey without squashing it. Remove any feather quills and fat from the bird and stuff both the crop and body.

■ Mix the tarragon into the butter and smear the breast and legs well with it. Sprinkle the turkey with freshly ground black pepper and put in the roasting tin.

■ Bring the stock, or mixture of stock, cider or wine, to the boil and pour over the turkey, until there is about 4 cm (1½ inches) liquid around the bird. Cover loosely with foil. Roast at 200°C (400°F) mark 6 near the bottom of the oven for 30 minutes. Lower the oven temperature to 180°C (350°F) mark 4 and continue cooking for 20 minutes for every 0.5 kg (1 lb) weight of bird.

■ After about 1½ hours, lift out the turkey, take off foil and baste well, adding a little more liquid if needed. Replace the foil and put the bird back in the oven the opposite way round, to ensure even cooking. Towards the end, test periodically and lower the heat if necessary; every carcass varies in shape and size, so it is hard to be precise about times.

■ When the turkey is cooked, put on to a warmed serving dish and keep hot. To make the gravy, pour or spoon off any excess fat from the roasting tin juices. Transfer the juices to a saucepan on the top of the stove and boil until reduced by half.

8 SERVINGS		10 SERVINGS	
kcals	435	kcals	345
kJ	1810	kJ	1450
CHO	Negligible	CHO	Negligible
Fibre	0	Fibre	0

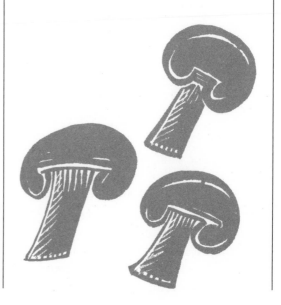

Djej Matisha Mesla

THIS EXCITING CHICKEN DISH which comes from a great centre of the Moorish-Andalusian culture, called Tetuan, in North Morocco makes a splendid party dish. The original recipe calls for a local very dark honey as an ingredient, but in this adaptation for diabetics I have used instead some sultanas or raisins, which give a very pleasing result. It is best if the marinating can be started the day before.

INGREDIENTS
1.6 kg (3½ lb) chicken, jointed
15 ml (1 tbsp) oil
1 medium onion, skinned and grated
300 ml (½ pint) chicken stock
700 g (1½ lb) ripe tomatoes, skinned and chopped
15 ml (1 tbsp) tomato purée
2.5 ml (½ tsp) ground cinnamon
25 g (1 oz) sultanas or raisins
25 g (1 oz) almonds or sesame seeds, roasted
For the marinade
pinch of ground turmeric
pinch of ground ginger
2 garlic cloves, skinned and crushed
salt and freshly ground black pepper
15 ml (1 tbsp) oil
SERVES 6

■ Wipe the chicken joints well and remove any lumps of fat. For the marinade, put the turmeric and ginger in a bowl with the garlic, salt and pepper, then mix in the oil, stirring vigorously to blend all together. Rub the mixture well into the chicken. Leave for at least 4 hours or, preferably, overnight, in a cool place.

■ When marinated, put the chicken, oil, grated onion and stock into a flameproof casserole. Bring to the boil and simmer, uncovered, for 10 minutes.

■ Add the tomatoes, tomato purée, cinnamon and a little more salt. Mix well and cook over a fairly high heat, turning from time to time, until the chicken is tender, about 25–30 minutes, making sure that the bottom does not catch. When most of the liquid has evaporated and the chicken is cooked, stir in the cinnamon and sultanas. Reduce the heat to low and sprinkle over the roasted almonds or sesame seeds. Serve with boiled brown or white rice.

6 SERVINGS	
kcals	265
kJ	1115
CHO	10 g
Fibre	3 g

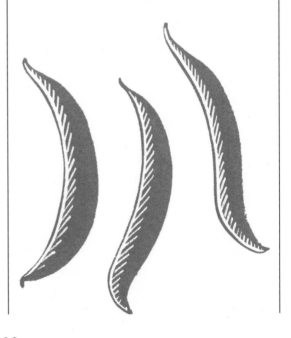

Pheasant with Celery and Cream

THIS RECIPE IS ONE which works well, too, with older birds.

INGREDIENTS
100 g (4 oz) butter or margarine
1 pheasant, well hung, plucked and cleaned
2 rashers bacon, derinded and diced
15 ml (1 tbsp) flour
300 ml (½ pint) chicken stock
pinch of dried tarragon
15 ml (1 tbsp) chopped fresh parsley
150 ml (¼ pint) red wine
salt and freshly ground black pepper
2 celery hearts, cut into rounds
1 egg yolk
300 ml (½ pint) single cream
SERVES 2 – 3

▮ Melt the butter in an ovenproof casserole on the top of the stove and brown the pheasant all over. Lift out the pheasant and brown the bacon just a little, then shake over the flour and allow to brown slightly. Add the stock, herbs and wine and season to taste.

▮ Put the pheasant back in the casserole and cover. Simmer slowly at 180°C (350°F) mark 4 for 30 minutes. Add the celery, cover and continue braising for another 30 minutes or until a thigh, pricked with a fork, gives out brown juice. Lift the bird on to a warmed serving dish and keep hot while preparing the sauce.

▮ Mix the egg yolk with the cream and beat slightly, then add a little of the hot stock to it, stirring well in. Gradually add the cream mixture to the rest of the juices in the casserole. Heat on the top of the stove, but do not reboil or the sauce will curdle. When thickened slightly, taste and adjust seasoning. Arrange the celery with the bacon around the pheasant and pour over some of the sauce, serving the rest in a warmed sauceboat.

2 SERVINGS		3 SERVINGS	
kcals	1400	kcals	1025
kJ	5860	kJ	4295
CHO	Negligible	CHO	Negligible
Fibre	0	Fibre	0

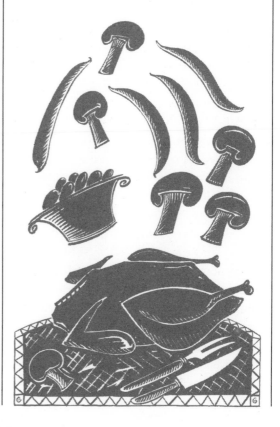

Wild Duck with Mustard Sauce

USE A MILD, French made, Dijon mustard for this dish, not a hot mustard.

INGREDIENTS
1.1–1.4 kg (2½–3 lb) wild duck
salt and freshly ground black pepper
25 g (1 oz) butter or margarine
duck's liver
15 ml (1 tbsp) oil
1 medium onion, skinned and chopped
150 ml (¼ pint) dry red wine
juice of ½ lemon or orange
grated rind of 1 lemon or orange
10 ml (2 tsp) Dijon mustard
SERVES 3

■ Season the bird inside and out and prick the skin of the breast slightly all over with a fine pronged fork. Put into a roasting tin. Roast at 190°C (375°F) mark 5 for 40 minutes.

■ While the duck is roasting, heat 15 g (½ oz) of the butter in a pan and sauté the duck liver. Put the liver and pan juices into a bowl and mash the liver into a paste. Put the remaining butter and the oil into the pan and soften the onion but do not allow it to colour. Add the red wine, bring to the boil and simmer for 5 minutes. Lower the heat and add the mashed liver and the remainder of the ingredients. Stir well and heat through but do not boil. Keep hot.

■ Carve the duck into portions and place on a warmed serving dish. Pour a little of the sauce over and serve the rest separately in a warmed sauceboat.

3 SERVINGS	
kcals	395
kJ	1645
CHO	Negligible
Fibre	0

Pigeon Breast Casserole

PIGEON BREASTS CAN BE FOUND at good poulterers and are an economical buy. They are easier to cook and serve than the whole bird and make a delicious rich-tasting casserole.

INGREDIENTS
8 large pigeon breasts
2 rashers streaky bacon, derinded and chopped
2 medium onions, skinned and sliced
3 medium carrots, scraped and sliced
300 ml (½ pint) beef stock
For the marinade
30 ml (2 tbsp) olive or sunflower oil
10 ml (2 tsp) red wine vinegar
pinch of finely chopped rosemary
1 garlic clove, skinned and chopped
SERVES 4

■ Put the oil, vinegar, rosemary, garlic and a pinch of black pepper into a dish. Add the pigeon breasts, turning to coat them all over. Cover loosely and leave in a cool place for 2–4 hours, turning once.

■ Fry the bacon in a non-stick pan until the fat runs out, but do not let it get too crisp. Add 15 ml (1 tbsp) of the strained

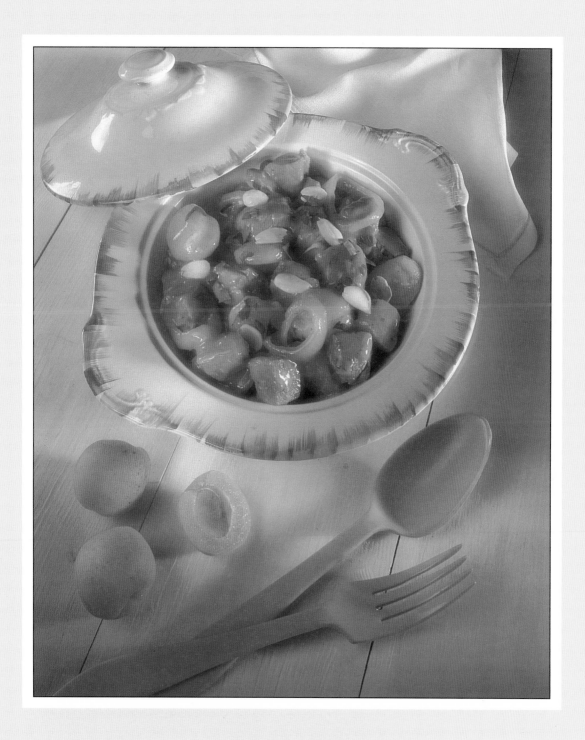

Pork with Apricots (page 78)

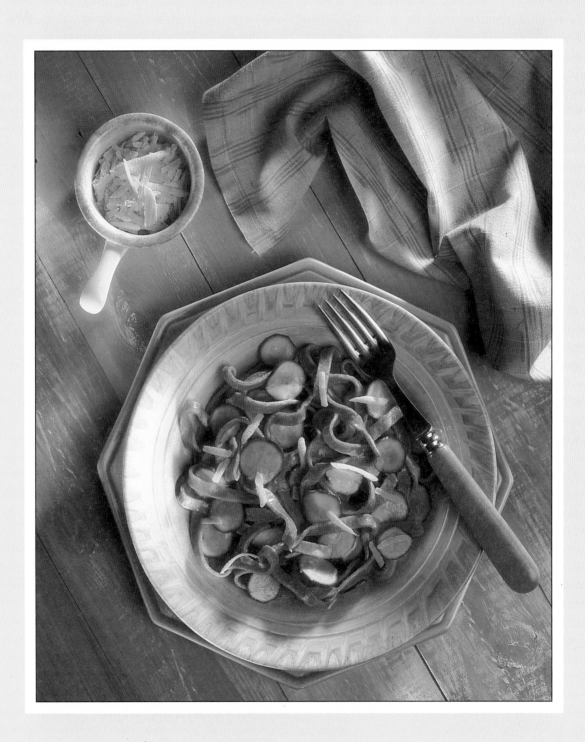

Pasta con le Zucchine (page 89)

marinade to the bacon and bring to the boil. Add the pigeon breasts and quickly fry them on both sides. Transfer to an ovenproof casserole, keeping the oil in the pan. Soften the vegetables in the oil and add to the casserole. Pour over the remaining marinade and the stock and season.

◼ Cover and cook at 180°C (350°F) mark 4 for about 1 hour or until tender.

4 SERVINGS	
kcals	590
kJ	2465
CHO	5 g
Fibre	2 g

Pigeon Breasts with Orange

AFTER MARINATING, frying the pigeon breasts provides a very quick and easy method.

INGREDIENTS
8 pigeon breasts
15 ml (1 tbsp) seasoned flour
25 g (1 oz) butter or margarine
juice of 1 orange
30 ml (2 tbsp) dry red wine
rind of $\frac{1}{2}$ orange, cut in julienne strips
For the marinade
30 ml (2 tbsp) oil
10 ml (2 tsp) red wine vinegar
5 ml (1 tsp) finely chopped fresh rosemary
1 garlic clove, skinned and chopped
SERVES 4

◼ Mix the marinade ingredients together in a dish and turn the breasts in it. Cover loosely and leave for 2–4 hours, turning the breasts once half way through.

◼ After marinating, lift out the breasts and roll them lightly in the seasoned flour. Heat the butter in a pan and quickly fry the breasts all over. Add the orange juice, boil and mix well with the pan juices. Add the red wine, stir again and simmer for 5 minutes.

◼ Meanwhile, blanch the orange rind strips for 2 minutes in boiling water and drain well. Put the pigeon breasts into a warmed serving dish, pour the pan juices over and garnish with the orange strips scattered on top.

4 SERVINGS	
kcals	465
kJ	1940
CHO	5 g
Fibre	0

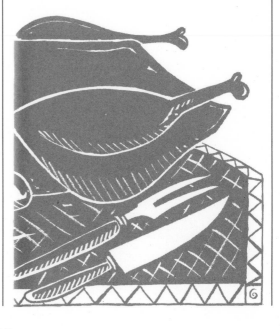

VENISON

IF YOU HAVE NEVER tasted venison, you have missed one of the greatest culinary delights. It is always very lean and, when properly prepared, tender and full of flavour. In addition, when we recall that it is also antibiotic and hormone free, you will see why I think so highly of it.

All game, and venison is no exception, profits from being marinated, not only to increase its tenderness but to enhance its flavour, while the marinade also serves as the basis for a superb sauce. The most traditional marinade is made with a little dry red wine, olive oil, herbs such as rosemary and parsley, spices such as all-spice corns and peppercorns, garlic and a sliced carrot. You can use a dry cider in place of the wine or, indeed, a dry home-made wine. The meat should be put into the marinade and turned from time to time, for 1–3 days, depending on the temperature of your cool larder. Marinating venison should never be attempted in the refrigerator. Even in the winter time, it is wise to cover with a screen to keep off any dust, insects or flies.

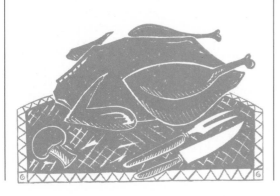

Venison Steaks with Orange

VENISON STEAKS SHOULD BE SLICED thinly from the leg and pounded between grease-proof paper before marinating.

INGREDIENTS
4 venison steaks, pounded
15 ml (1 tbsp) olive oil
15 ml (1 tbsp) seasoned flour
60 ml (4 tbsp) dry red wine
juice of 2 oranges
salt and freshly ground black pepper

SERVES 4

▮ Brush the venison steaks with half the olive oil, then lightly roll them in the seasoned flour. Heat the remaining oil in a pan and fry the steaks very quickly on both sides. Take the steaks out and keep them hot.

▮ Add the wine and orange juice to the pan, bring to the boil and boil rapidly for about 1 minute to reduce, stirring vigorously. Taste and adjust seasoning if necessary. Pour the sauce over the steaks and serve at once.

4 SERVINGS	
kcals	275
kJ	1155
CHO	5 g
Fibre	0

VARIATION

INSTEAD OF DRY RED WINE, 60 ml (4 tbsp) crème fraiche (cultivated soured cream) can be stirred well into the pan juices and poured over the steaks.

Roast Venison

CHOOSE THE LEG, saddle or shoulder joint for roasting.

INGREDIENTS

1.8–2.3 kg (4–5 lb) joint of venison

4–6 rashers streaky bacon, derinded

10 ml (2 tsp) finely chopped fresh rosemary

freshly ground black pepper

pinch of ground cinnamon

pinch of ground ginger

5 ml (1 tsp) salt

10 ml (2 tsp) lemon juice

15 ml (1 tbsp) diabetic redcurrant jelly (optional)

15 g ($\frac{1}{2}$ oz) butter or margarine

2 cooking apples, cored but unpeeled, cut in rings

For the marinade

300 ml ($\frac{1}{2}$ pint) dry red wine or dry cider

1 large garlic clove, skinned and chopped

30–45 ml (2–3 tbsp) olive oil

large sprig of rosemary

large sprig of parsley

4–6 whole allspice corns or juniper berries, slightly crushed

6 black peppercorns

2 bay leaves

1 medium carrot, scraped and sliced

3 shallots or 1 medium onion, skinned and chopped

SERVES 8 – 10

■ Mix the marinade ingredients together in a dish. Add the venison and marinate for 1–3 days, turning from time to time, in a cool larder.

■ Lift out the venison, pat dry with absorbent kitchen paper and put into a roasting tin. Lay the rashers of bacon over the joint, sprinkle over the rosemary and pepper. Boil the marinade with the cinnamon, ginger and salt. Through a strainer, pour half of this over the joint and reserve the rest. Cover the joint loosely with foil.

■ Cook at 200°C (400°F) mark 6 for 30 minutes per 0.5 kg (1 lb), basting from time to time. If it is a very large joint, 2.7 kg (6 lb) or over, you can reduce the cooking time to 20 minutes per 0.5 kg (1 lb). To brown the top, take off the foil for the last 30 minutes. When cooked, remove to a warmed serving dish and keep hot.

■ Strain the juices from the roasting tin into a saucepan, large enough to take the remainder of the marinade, also strained. Bring to the boil, add the lemon juice and redcurrant jelly and boil to reduce, stirring continuously. Taste for seasoning and adjust if needed. Finally, add half the butter to give the finished sauce a glaze. Transfer to a warmed sauceboat and keep hot.

■ Heat the remaining butter in a pan and lightly fry the apple rings. Garnish the joint with the fried apple rings and serve accompanied by the sauce.

8 SERVINGS		10 SERVINGS	
kcals	500	kcals	400
kJ	2090	kJ	1670
CHO	5 g	CHO	5 g
Fibre	0	Fibre	0

MEAT

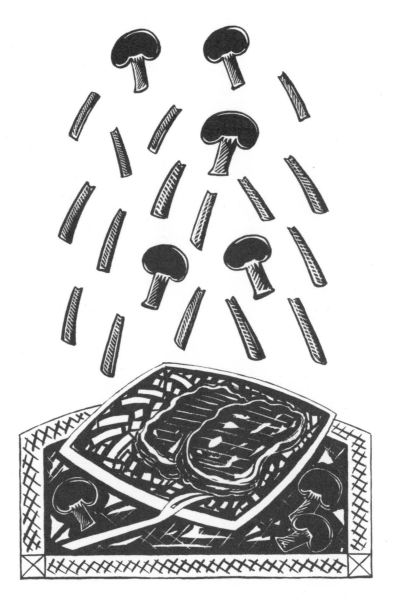

MEAT IS NOT ONLY an expensive item in most households, it is also, in general, the worst cooked food eaten. Many joints are over-cooked, thus depriving the consumer of much of the vitamin content as well as spoiling the flavour. It really is well worth taking proper care in the roasting of meat, so that the good juices are retained and one is not left with a joint as dry and tough as a block of mahogany! The over-cooking of meat is also a frequent cause of chronic indigestion, as the human digestive enzymes find it hard to tackle really incinerated and dried up meat. The avoidance of this is particularly important to diabetics and they, at least, should make sure that such unsuitable food does not appear on their tables. Remember too, that under-roasted meat can always be cooked a little more, but over-roasting is a complete waste of time and money. If circumstances are such that you do not have the time to plan and attend to roasting, it is far safer to plan for a casserole or stew, or use a slow cooker. Perhaps cheaper cuts are a little more trouble to prepare but, once done, they can be frozen for use when you do not have the time to prepare them.

Pork is, of course, an exception, always needing to be cooked until it is no longer pink, even at the very centre or next to the bone.

Beef Casserole with Celery and Walnuts

STEWING OR BRAISING STEAK are equally successful to use in this flavoursome casserole.

INGREDIENTS
30 ml (2 tbsp) oil
1 kg (2¼ lb) rib steak, trimmed and cubed
2 medium onions, skinned and chopped
3 garlic cloves, skinned and crushed
15 ml (1 tbsp) flour
150 ml (¼ pint) dry red wine
300 ml (½ pint) beef stock
salt and freshly ground black pepper
4–5 celery stalks, trimmed and chopped
50 g (2 oz) walnuts, chopped
rind of 1 orange, cut into julienne strips, blanched
SERVES 4

■ Heat the oil in a pan and seal and brown the meat cubes on the outside, working with a few cubes at a time so that the oil remains hot. Remove them to a casserole as they brown. Add the onions

and garlic to the pan and sauté until lightly browned. Sprinkle in the flour and continue cooking for 2–3 minutes.

■ Pour in the wine and bring to the boil, stirring vigorously to avoid the flour lumping. Add the stock, return to the boil and simmer until the volume is reduced by half. Season to taste and pour over the beef.

■ Cover and cook at 180°C (350°F) mark 4 for 1½ hours or until the meat is tender when tested with a fork. For the last 15 minutes of cooking, add the celery, walnuts and orange rind strips. Serve with new potatoes or boiled brown rice.

4 SERVINGS	
kcals	610
kJ	2535
CHO	5 g
Fibre	2 g

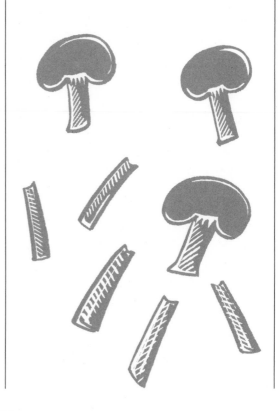

Beef and Ginger Casserole

THIS DISH CAN BE COOKED ahead of time and will improve in flavour when re-heated, on top of the stove or in the oven.

INGREDIENTS
30 ml (2 tbsp) oil
3 bay leaves
900 g (2 lb) lean stewing beef, cubed
1 large onion, skinned and sliced
15 ml (1 tbsp) flour
pinch of dried marjoram
600 ml (1 pint) beef stock
30 ml (2 tbsp) peeled and chopped fresh root ginger
salt and freshly ground black pepper
SERVES 4

■ Heat the oil in a flameproof casserole on the top of the stove and put in the bay leaves, covering for a moment in case they splash as they crisp. Add the beef cubes, a few at a time, and seal and brown them. When browned, add the onion and soften until golden. Shake in the flour and marjoram and cook for 2 minutes. Add the beef stock, stirring well to avoid lumping, bring to the boil, add the ginger and season to taste.

■ Cover and cook at 190°C (375°F) mark 5 for 1½–2 hours. Check at least once that the liquid is not drying up and add a little stock or water if needed.

4 SERVINGS	
kcals	470
kJ	1965
CHO	5 g
Fibre	1 g

Beef with Peppers

A MOST ATTRACTIVE, quick stir-fry dish which can easily be adapted for a single person or for a large party, by just cutting down or increasing the amounts to scale—not something that works with every recipe, but it does with this one. Don't forget though, if preparing for a party, to make sure that your wok or frying pan is capacious enough to handle the amount without spilling over.

INGREDIENTS
700 g (1½ lb) beef topside, sliced very thinly and pounded
30 ml (2 tbsp) vegetable oil
2 garlic cloves, skinned and finely chopped
2 medium onions, skinned and thinly sliced
1 ripe red pepper, cored, deseeded and sliced in thin strips
1 ripe yellow pepper, cored, deseeded and sliced in thin strips
For the marinade
15 ml (1 tbsp) vegetable oil
15 ml (1 tbsp) dry sherry or dry rice wine
30 ml (2 tbsp) soy sauce
5 ml (1 tsp) sesame oil
SERVES 4 – 5

■ Cut the beef into short strips. Mix the marinade ingredients well together in a bowl. Put in the meat strips and stir thoroughly to ensure that the meat is coated all over with the marinade. Leave, covered, in a cool place for 1 hour.

■ Heat 15 ml (1 tbsp) of the oil in a wok or large frying pan and stir-fry the garlic until soft. Add the onions and stir-fry until just golden, then add the pepper strips and continue stir-frying for 2 minutes but do not let the onions take more colour. Remove the vegetables from the wok or pan and keep them hot.

■ Heat the remaining oil and, when really hot, brown the beef quickly, keeping the strips from sticking together by vigorous use of a wooden spoon or spatula. Return the vegetables to the wok or pan and mix thoroughly. Serve immediately with boiled brown rice or with cooked dried beans (see pages 84–92).

4 SERVINGS		5 SERVINGS	
kcals	425	kcals	340
kJ	1775	kJ	1415
CHO	5 g	CHO	Negligible
Fibre	1 g	Fibre	Negligible

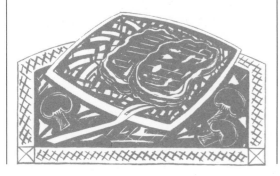

Veal with Cucumber

IN THIS RECIPE, the veal needs to be beaten until it is flat and thin.

INGREDIENTS
1 medium cucumber, peeled
salt and freshly ground black pepper or crushed green pepper
100 g (4 oz) butter
4 fillet of veal slices, beaten
45 ml (3 tbsp) single cream
15 ml (1 tbsp) finely chopped fresh parsley, to garnish
SERVES 4

■ Cut the cucumber into 2.5 cm (1 inch) sections. Simmer in lightly salted water for 10 minutes, then drain and keep hot.

■ Heat 50 g (2 oz) of the butter in a pan and quickly seal and brown the veal on both sides, then take out and keep hot. Scrape the pan well with a wooden spoon or spatula to lift the meat residue, then mix in the cream and seasoning. Boil for a moment to thicken, then draw to the side and add the rest of the butter, a small piece at a time, mixing well.

■ Finally add the cooked cucumber pieces and heat, coating them with the sauce. Lay the veal slices on top, cover and simmer gently for 15 minutes. Serve at once, garnished with the parsley.

4 SERVINGS	
kcals	400
kJ	1655
CHO	Negligible
Fibre	0

Paupiettes de Boeuf

PAUPIETTES ARE THIN SLICES OF BEEF rolled around stuffing.

INGREDIENTS

8 very thin slices of beef silverside, 75 g (2–3 oz) each, pounded
30 ml (2 tbsp) oil
400 g (14 oz) tomatoes, skinned, deseeded and liquidised or equal quantity of canned, drained and liquidised
30 ml (2 tbsp) dry red wine
150 ml (¼ pint) beef stock
pinch of dried oregano
1 green or yellow pepper, cored, deseeded, sliced and sautéed
For the stuffing
30 ml (2 tbsp) Dijon mustard
8 rashers streaky bacon, derinded
8 medium mushrooms, sliced
freshly ground black pepper
SERVES 4

▌ Trim any fat from the silverside slices and lay them flat on a working surface. Spread each slice with a thin layer of mustard, lay a rasher of bacon on each, then some of the mushrooms. Grind a little black pepper over each and roll up, securing with string.

▌ Heat the oil in a pan and seal and brown each roll all over. Place them in an ovenproof casserole, but retain the pan juices in the pan. Add the liquidised tomatoes, the wine and stock to the pan. Bring to the boil, scatter over the oregano and stir well in. Pour the sauce over the paupiettes and cover.

▌ Cook at 180°C (350°F) mark 4 for 1½–2 hours or until the meat is tender when tested with a fork. About 20 minutes before serving, remove the string, scatter the pepper around, cover again and finish cooking.

4 SERVINGS	
kcals	665
kJ	2760
CHO	5 g
Fibre	0

Il Garafolato

THIS IS A ROMAN BEEF STEW with cloves, which is deliciously warming and full of flavour. It takes its name from the Italian word for clove which is *garofano*. This dish can be made equally well in a covered flameproof casserole simmered very gently on the top of the stove for the same length of time.

INGREDIENTS

30 ml (2 tbsp) olive oil
1.1 kg (2½ lb) lean stewing beef, cubed
1 large onion, skinned and sliced
2 garlic cloves, skinned and crushed
1 small head of celery, trimmed and chopped
10 ml (2 tsp) chopped fresh parsley
1 cm (½ inch) cinnamon stick
pinch of freshly grated nutmeg
6 whole cloves
3 large ripe tomatoes, skinned and chopped, or canned, drained
150 ml (¼ pint) dry red wine
300 ml (½ pint) beef stock
salt and freshly ground black pepper
SERVES 4 – 5

■ Heat a third of the oil in a frying pan and seal and brown the meat cubes quickly, a few at a time. Transfer them to a flameproof casserole as they brown. Add another third of the oil to the pan and soften the onion and garlic but do not brown. Transfer to the casserole.

■ Add the remaining third of the oil to the pan and soften the celery, adding the parsley and spices to the pan. Cook for a further 1 minute, then add the tomatoes and wine. Bring to the boil, stir well and simmer for 2 minutes. Transfer the contents of the pan to the casserole together with the stock. Stir well, season to taste and cover.

■ Cook at 170°C (325°F) mark 3 for 2 hours. Half an hour before the end of the cooking time, uncover, stir, and add a little water if it has become too dry.

4 SERVINGS	
kcals	545
kJ	2270
CHO	5 g
Fibre	2 g

5 SERVINGS	
kcals	435
kJ	1815
CHO	5 g
Fibre	2 g

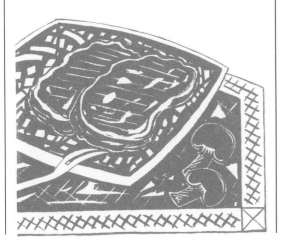

Steak au Poivre

THIS IS A DISH that cannot be kept waiting, even for a king!

INGREDIENTS
30 ml (2 tbsp) black or green peppercorns, coarsely crushed
4 beef steaks, fillet or sirloin, 175 g (6 oz) each
15 g (½ oz) butter or margarine
30 ml (2 tbsp) brandy or dry sherry (optional)
SERVES 4

■ Press the coarsely crushed peppercorns into both sides of each steak, so that the meat is well covered. Heat the butter until very hot in a heavy pan and fry the steaks carefully on both sides, being careful to dislodge as little pepper as possible when turning. It is important that the pan is hot enough for the steaks to sizzle loudly when put in, they should be cooked as quickly as possible so that they take colour on the outside while remaining rare on the inside, if you like them that way. If preferred well done, just cook the steaks a little longer. To test if the steaks are ready, make a small nick with the point of a sharp knife.

■ When they are done to your liking, if using warm the brandy or sherry in a ladle, ignite and pour over. When the flames have died down, serve at once on warmed plates with a fair distribution of the pan juices on each.

4 SERVINGS	
kcals	495
kJ	2040
CHO	0
Fibre	0

73

Loin of Lamb with Apple and Ginger Stuffing

SPINACH MAKES A VERY GOOD VEGETABLE to serve with this dish.

INGREDIENTS

1.4 kg (3 lb) loin of lamb, skinned and boned

2 garlic cloves, skinned and sliced

salt and freshly ground black pepper

300 ml ($\frac{1}{2}$ pint) dry cider

For the stuffing

2 medium cooking apples, peeled, cored and thinly sliced

juice of 1 lemon

10 ml (2 tsp) peeled and finely chopped fresh root ginger

SERVES 5 – 6

■ For the stuffing, put the apple, lemon juice and ginger in a saucepan over a gentle heat. Cover and simmer gently until the apple is just soft. Allow to cool.

■ Lay the boned loin of lamb, outside down, on a flat board. Spoon the apple mixture along the centre, roll up and tie with cooking string. With a sharp knife, prick the outside of the joint and insert the garlic slices. Season.

■ Place the joint in a roasting tin. Roast at 200°C (400°F) mark 6 for 30 minutes. Bring the cider to the boil and pour over the joint. Reduce the oven temperature to 180°C (350°F) mark 4 and roast for another 40 minutes, basting often.

■ Test with a fork to check the meat is cooked. Remove from the oven, put on a warmed serving dish and keep hot. Pour away the fat from the roasting tin juices.

Boil the juices on top of the stove until slightly reduced. Serve in a sauceboat to accompany the joint.

5 SERVINGS		6 SERVINGS	
kcals	330	kcals	275
kJ	1385	kJ	1155
CHO	5 g	CHO	5 g
Fibre	1 g	Fibre	1 g

Arabian Lamb

THIS IS ONE OF THOSE DISHES that actually improve if made the day before and re-heated. It makes an admirable party dish, for which the quantities can be doubled to serve 10. Do not freeze this dish for more than about a week or two at the most.

INGREDIENTS

30 ml (2 tbsp) vegetable oil

900 g (2 lb) lean boned lamb, cubed

3 medium onions, skinned and sliced

30 ml (2 tbsp) ground coriander

30 ml (2 tbsp) ground cumin

5 ml (1 tsp) ground ginger

1.25 ml ($\frac{1}{4}$ tsp) ground turmeric

1.25 ml ($\frac{1}{4}$ tsp) ground chilli

15 ml (1 tbsp) tomato purée

15 ml (1 tbsp) flour

600 ml (1 pint) lamb or chicken stock

225 g (8 oz) tomatoes, skinned, quartered and deseeded

75 g (3 oz) sultanas

salt and freshly ground black pepper

SERVES 5

▌ Heat the oil in a flameproof casserole. When really hot, seal and brown the meat cubes, a few at a time. Take them out as they brown and keep hot. Lower the heat and soften the onions but do not let them brown. Add all the spices and cook for a further 2 minutes. Stir in the tomato purée and cook for 1 minute, stirring well. Add the flour and cook for 2 minutes more, continuing to stir.

▌ Pour in the stock, a little at a time, stirring vigorously to prevent lumping, as the contents of the pan return to the boil. Add the tomatoes, sultanas and the meat, mix well and season to taste.

▌ Cover and cook at 170°C (325°F) mark 3 for about 2 hours or until the meat is tender when tested with a fork.

5 SERVINGS	
kcals	425
kJ	1785
CHO	15 g
Fibre	2 g

VARIATION

AN EVEN BETTER FLAVOUR can be obtained by using mutton instead of lamb, increasing the cooking time by a further 40 minutes.

Lamb Boulangère

A CLASSICAL FRENCH TREATMENT of lamb. If the shoulder is used, it must be trimmed of fat, then boned and rolled. Do not attempt to freeze this dish.

INGREDIENTS
1.4–1.6 kg (3–3½ lb) half leg or whole shoulder of lamb
2 garlic cloves, skinned and sliced
6 small sprigs of rosemary
salt and freshly ground black pepper or crushed green pepper
30 ml (2 tbsp) olive oil
700 g (1½ lb) potatoes, peeled and thickly sliced
450 g (1 lb) onions, skinned and sliced in rings
300 ml (½ pint) lamb stock
SERVES 4 – 6

▌ With a small, sharp knife, make little nicks in the skin of the joint and insert the garlic slices and rosemary sprigs, distributing them evenly over the surface of the joint. Rub the skin with salt and black or green pepper and brush it over with 15 ml (1 tbsp) of the oil.

▌ Use a little of the remaining oil to grease an ovenproof baking dish, then layer it with the potato and onion slices, in alternate layers, seasoning them as you do so. Pour over the stock and the remainder of the oil. Lay the joint on top.

▌ Roast at 180°C (350°F) mark 4 for 1½ hours. If you find that your oven is making the lamb or the vegetables too brown on the outside, put foil over the dish, dull side down, for the remainder of the cooking time.

4 SERVINGS		6 SERVINGS	
kcals	480	kcals	320
kJ	2030	kJ	1355
CHO	45 g	CHO	30 g
Fibre	5 g	Fibre	3 g

Butterfly Leg of Lamb with Herbs

6 SERVINGS		8 SERVINGS	
kcals	355	kcals	265
kJ	1490	kJ	1120
CHO	0	CHO	0
Fibre	0	Fibre	0

THIS IS A REALLY GOOD high summer dish, when a plentiful variety of fresh herbs are available. It is best to marinate the lamb overnight, covered, in a cool place. Your butcher will bone the leg of lamb for you.

INGREDIENTS
1.8 kg (4 lb) leg of lamb, boned
salt
For the marinade
15 ml (1 tbsp) finely chopped fresh parsley
10 ml (2 tsp) finely chopped fresh marjoram
5 ml (1 tsp) finely chopped fresh rosemary
5 ml (1 tsp) finely chopped fresh lemon thyme
2 garlic cloves, skinned and finely chopped
150 ml ($\frac{1}{4}$ pint) dry red wine or dry cider
15 ml (1 tbsp) olive oil
10 ml (2 tsp) freshly squeezed lemon juice
freshly ground black pepper
SERVES 6 – 8

■ Trim all excess fat from the lamb and spread it out flat, inside down, in a roasting tin. Mix together all the ingredients for the marinade. Pour over the joint and leave, covered, in a cool place to marinate for 24 hours, turning several times.

■ Next day sprinkle the lamb with salt, leaving the marinade in the roasting tin. Roast, uncovered, at 180°C (350°F) mark 4 for 1½ hours, basting with the marinade 2–3 times during the last 30 minutes.

■ Place the joint on a warmed serving dish and keep hot. Boil the roasting tin juices until reduced by half. Serve as an accompanying sauce in a sauceboat.

Lamb and Aubergine Spicy Casserole

ACCOMPANY THIS DELICIOUS SPICED LAMB dish with brown rice.

INGREDIENTS
1 large aubergine, about 450 g (1 lb), peeled and cubed
15 ml (1 tbsp) salt
15 ml (1 tbsp) sunflower oil
700 g (1½ lb) cubed lamb, trimmed of fat
3 medium onions, skinned and finely chopped
freshly ground black pepper
2.5 ml ($\frac{1}{2}$ tsp) ground allspice
2.5 ml ($\frac{1}{2}$ tsp) ground cinnamon
2.5 ml ($\frac{1}{2}$ tsp) caraway seeds
425 g (15 oz) can tomatoes and their juice
1 large garlic clove, skinned and crushed
300 ml ($\frac{1}{2}$ pint) lamb stock
SERVES 4 – 5

■ Put the aubergine into a colander, sprinkle with salt and set aside.

■ Heat the oil in a large frying pan and, when really hot, seal and brown the lamb cubes, a few at a time. Remove them from the pan as they brown. When all are browned, reduce the heat.

■ Drain the aubergine cubes well and pat dry with absorbent kitchen paper. Soften them gently in the pan with the onions, without browning. Return the browned lamb cubes to the pan and add the spices. Cook for 1 minute, raising the heat a little if needed, then add the tomatoes, garlic and stock.

■ Bring quickly to the boil, then cover and simmer for about 1 hour until the meat is tender, stirring from time to time. Just before serving, check the seasoning and adjust if needed.

4 SERVINGS		5 SERVINGS	
kcals	355	kcals	285
kJ	1485	kJ	1190
CHO	10 g	CHO	5 g
Fibre	5 g	Fibre	4 g

Marinated Lamb Steaks

OTHER THAN ON A CHARCOAL GRILL, to cook any kind of steak well, you must have either a very hot, heavy pan or a heavy cast iron grilling plate mounted on a gas burner. Alternatively, use an electric infra-red grill of sufficient size and capacity to be able to cope with the quick grilling speed that is necessary for good results. But the important point is that, whichever method you use, there must be enough rapidly available heat immediately to seal in the meat juices. Where the grilling surfaces come into contact with both the upper and lower surfaces of the steaks, it is vital to remove any bones that could prevent an even contact.

INGREDIENTS
4 lamb steaks, cut from the top of the leg, each 175 g (6 oz)
coarse salt
thick lemon wedges, to serve
For the marinade
30 ml (2 tbsp) olive oil
15 ml (1 tbsp) red wine vinegar
5 ml (1 tsp) finely chopped fresh rosemary
5 ml (1 tsp) finely chopped fresh tarragon
5 ml (1 tsp) ground coriander
1 small garlic clove, skinned and finely chopped
freshly ground black pepper or crushed green pepper
SERVES 4

■ Mix the oil and vinegar well together. Put the steaks in a shallow dish and pour over the marinade, turning them so that the marinade reaches both sides. Scatter half the herbs, the coriander and garlic over them and give a good grind or sprinkle of pepper. Turn the steaks again, scatter over the remainder of the herbs and garlic and give another grind or sprinkle of pepper. Leave the lamb steaks to marinate for a few hours, turning from time to time.

■ Heat the pan or infra-red grill until it is very hot. Quickly put the steaks on to it and grill for 3–5 minutes on each side, depending on whether you like your steaks rare or well done. Just before serving, scatter the meat with a little coarse salt and serve with wedges of lemon.

4 SERVINGS	
kcals	545
kJ	2290
CHO	0
Fibre	0

Moussaka

THIS IS A GOOD, all purpose dish which is ideal at all times of year, with either beef or lamb. At the time, if aubergines are too dear, it can be made with softened courgettes, peppers or cauliflower florets.

INGREDIENTS
700 g (1½ lb) aubergines, peeled and cubed
15 ml (1 tbsp) salt
60 ml (4 tbsp) oil
450 g (1 lb) lean minced lamb or beef
1 large onion, skinned and chopped
1 garlic clove, skinned and chopped
425 g (15 oz) can tomatoes, drained
freshly ground black pepper
1.25 ml (¼ tsp) ground cinnamon
1 egg, size 2
150 ml (¼ pint) milk
15 ml (1 tbsp) grated hard cheese
SERVES 4

■ Put the aubergine cubes into a colander, sprinkle well with salt and set aside for 30 minutes. Pat dry with absorbent kitchen paper.

■ Heat 30 ml (2 tbsp) of the oil in a frying pan and, when really hot, seal and brown the minced meat, a little at a time. Remove the mince as it browns and keep hot. Lower the heat and soften the onion and garlic in the pan but do not allow them to brown. Add the tomatoes and return the meat to the pan, bring to the boil and simmer for 10 minutes.

■ Meanwhile, heat the remainder of the oil in another pan and soften the aubergine cubes, without letting them take on any colour.

■ Layer the vegetables and meat alternately in an oiled ovenproof dish, giving a grind of pepper and a sprinkling of ground cinnamon to each layer, finishing with meat sauce. Beat the egg into the milk, pour over the top layer and scatter over the grated cheese. Bake at 180°C (350°F) mark 4 for 45 minutes until golden.

4 SERVINGS	
kcals	395
kJ	1665
CHO	10 g
Fibre	6 g

Pork with Apricots

DRIED APRICOTS are used in this spicy pork dish.

INGREDIENTS
30 ml (2 tbsp) oil
1.4–1.8 kg (3–4 lb) shoulder of pork, trimmed, boned and cubed
4 medium onions, skinned and sliced
2 garlic cloves, skinned and chopped
5 ml (1 tsp) ground ginger
5 ml (1 tsp) ground coriander
5 ml (1 tsp) ground cumin
150 ml (¼ pint) dry white wine or chicken stock
225 g (8 oz) dried apricots, soaked for 4 hours in water to cover
salt and freshly ground black pepper or crushed green pepper
50 g (2 oz) almonds, blanched and halved
chopped fresh parsley, to garnish
SERVES 6 – 8

■ Heat the oil in a large frying pan and, when it is really hot, seal and brown the meat cubes, a few at a time. Remove the meat from the pan as it browns and keep hot. When all the meat cubes are browned, lower the heat and soften the onions and garlic, without letting them take colour.

■ Pour away any excess fat from the pan and add the spices and wine, stirring vigorously to mix. Return the meat cubes to the pan, add three-quarters of the soaked apricots together with all of the soaking water. Cover and simmer for 45–55 minutes until the pork is tender. Season to taste.

■ Lightly brown the blanched, halved almonds in a hot dry pan, shaking them continuously. Chop and add the remaining apricots to the browned almonds. Heat through and use to garnish the dish with the parsley. Serve with boiled brown rice cooked with a pinch of saffron, if available.

6 SERVINGS		8 SERVINGS	
kcals	430	kcals	320
kJ	1790	kJ	1345
CHO	20 g	CHO	15 g
Fibre	11 g	Fibre	8 g

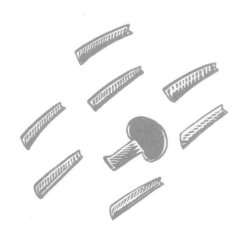

Savoy Pork Chops

APPLES COMPLEMENT PORK and here they are cooked with the chops.

INGREDIENTS
4 lean pork chops
30 ml (2 tbsp) oil
4 medium onions, skinned and sliced
4 medium to large cooking apples, peeled, cored and sliced
pinch of ground sage
pinch of dried tarragon
30 ml (2 tbsp) sultanas
300 ml (½ pint) chicken stock or dry cider
salt and freshly ground black pepper
SERVES 4

■ Trim the pork chops of any fat or gristle. Heat 15 ml (1 tbsp) of the oil in a non-stick frying pan and quickly seal and brown the chops on both sides. Lift them out and keep hot. Add the remainder of the oil and gently soften the onions without browning. Remove.

■ Soften the apples in the same way, lift out and keep them hot with the onions. Raise the heat a little, put the chops back into the pan and continue frying until cooked well through.

■ Pour off any excess oil and return the onion and apple to the pan, together with the herbs and sultanas. Mix well, then add the stock and simmer until the sauce thickens slightly and all the ingredients are well cooked. Season to taste.

4 SERVINGS	
kcals	315
kJ	1325
CHO	20 g
Fibre	4 g

Noisettes de Porc aux Pruneaux

THIS DELIGHTFUL DISH, from Tours in France, uses either prunes or plums. If using loin of pork, ask your butcher to roll and tie the pork for you. If he isn't very expert at this, it is better to use the pork fillets. It makes an excellent party dish for it does not spoil if your guests are late!

INGREDIENTS
12–16 prunes, soaked for 4 hours, or 450 g (1 lb) dark plums, stoned
300 ml (½ pint) dry white wine
pinch of ground cinnamon
1.1–1.4 kg (2½–3 lb) boned loin of pork, trimmed of fat, or 3 pork fillets, trimmed of fat
25 g (1 oz) flour
40–50 g (1½–2 oz) butter
150 ml (¼ pint) single cream
salt and freshly ground black pepper or crushed green pepper
10 ml (2 tsp) lemon juice
SERVES 6 – 8

■ Soak the prunes or plums in the wine for at least 4 hours or preferably overnight. If using prunes, stone them and return to the liquid. Cover and simmer for 30 minutes. If using plums, cover and simmer for 10 minutes. After cooking, set aside in the liquid.

■ Slice the rolled loin or pork fillets across 1 cm (½ inch) thick, to make the little rounds of meat the French call noisettes. Make sure all but the thinnest layer of fat on the outside is removed. Flour each slice, patting off any excess.

■ Heat the butter well in a non-stick pan and seal the noisettes, a few at a time, on both sides. Cook them until they cease to be pink in the middle but are only a light gold on the outside. Remove to a warmed serving dish and keep hot. If using the rolled loin, be sure to remove any pieces of string.

■ Heat the fruit in its liquid. Drain, keeping the liquid for the sauce, and arrange the fruit around the cooked noisettes. Add the fruit liquid to the frying pan, bring to the boil and simmer until reduced by half. Lower the heat, add the cream, mixing well, and bring almost to the boil. Do not boil or the cream will curdle. Taste for seasoning and adjust if necessary. Add the lemon juice and stir.

■ Pour the sauce over the pork and serve at once. Everything can be prepared to the point just before adding the cream. The dish can be kept hot for some time without spoiling if your guests are late. Do not finish the sauce until just before serving.

6 SERVINGS		8 SERVINGS	
kcals	410	kcals	305
kJ	1710	kJ	1280
CHO	10 g	CHO	10 g
Fibre	3 g	Fibre	2 g

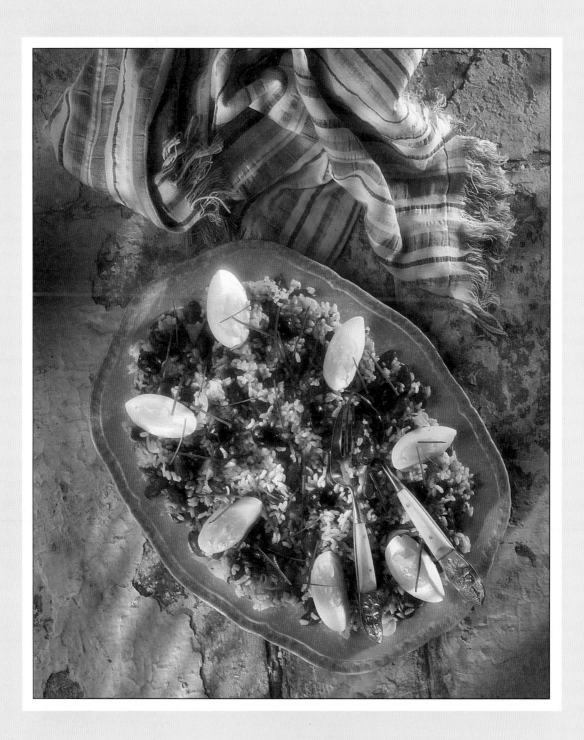

Spanish Rice (page 90)

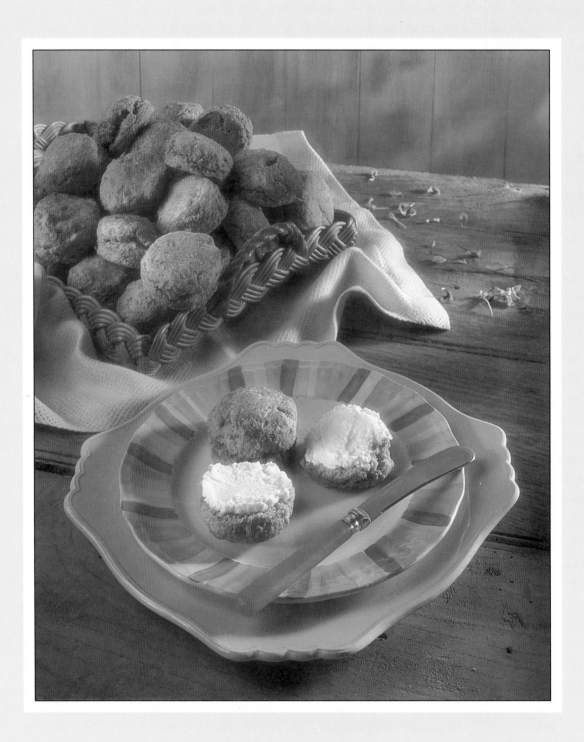

Wholemeal Apple Scones (page 122)

Ossi Buchi Milanese—Braised Veal Shin

IT IS ESSENTIAL first to find a butcher who will supply you with veal shin bones, filled with marrow and with quite a lot of meat still left around the bone. Your butcher will saw them to the appropriate lengths, 5–7.5 cm (2–3 inches). In Milan, this dish is always served with risotto Milanese, see page 88.

INGREDIENTS
4 veal shin bones, 225 g (8 oz) each
flour for dusting
45 ml (3 tbsp) olive oil or butter
1 medium onion, skinned and sliced
1 garlic clove, skinned and chopped
150 ml ($\frac{1}{4}$ pint) dry white wine
425 g (15 oz) can tomatoes
salt and freshly ground black pepper
To garnish
60 ml (4 tbsp) finely chopped fresh parsley
1 large garlic clove, skinned and finely chopped
finely grated rind of $\frac{1}{2}$ lemon
SERVES 4

■ Dust the sections of marrow bones with flour. Heat the oil in a large pan and carefully fry them, without disturbing the marrow in the bones. Lift out gently and transfer to an ovenproof dish, arranging them with the marrow upright.

■ In the same oil, soften the onion, without browning. Add the garlic and cook for 1 minute. Pour over the white wine, raise the heat and bring to the boil, then add the tomatoes and half the juice. Stir well and raise the heat if needed to allow the pan contents to reduce a little, then add the remaining juice, boiling fairly rapidly. Season to taste and pour over the shin bones.

■ Braise at 180°C (350°F) mark 4 for 1–1$\frac{1}{2}$ hours, reducing the oven temperature to 170°C (325°F) mark 3 if it appears to be cooking too fast.

■ Meanwhile prepare the garnish, which is called *Gremolata* in Milan. Mix together the parsley, garlic and lemon rind. Scatter over the tops of the veal bones and serve.

4 SERVINGS	
kcals	220
kJ	920
CHO	4 g
Fibre	2 g

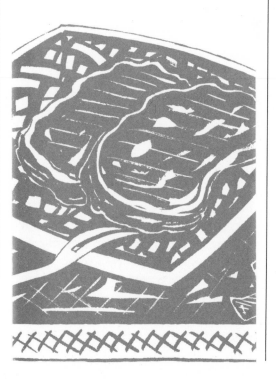

Mexican Pork Chops

THIS DISH MAKES ONE of the easiest and most delicious meals-in-one, as it need only be accompanied by a green salad. It can easily be adapted to serve more people by simply increasing the ingredients to the number you want. It is particularly good and nutritious when brown rice is used.

INGREDIENTS

4 lean pork chops, boned

5 ml (1 tsp) oil

1 large onion, skinned and sliced in rings

1 green pepper, cored, deseeded and sliced

100 g (4 oz) brown or white rice

1.25 ml ($\frac{1}{4}$ tsp) ground chilli

425 g (15 oz) can tomatoes

150 ml ($\frac{1}{4}$ pint) tomato juice

pinch of ground sage

5 ml (1 tsp) finely chopped fresh thyme

salt and freshly ground black pepper or crushed green pepper

SERVES 4

■ Trim off any remaining fat from the chops. Heat the oil in a non-stick frying pan and, when really hot, seal and brown the chops on both sides. Transfer them to the bottom of a flameproof casserole.

■ Reduce the heat in the pan and soften the onion and pepper, without letting them brown. Spoon them over the chops. Scatter the rice as evenly as possible over the contents of the casserole. Mix together the remaining ingredients and pour over the top.

■ Cover and bake at 180°C (350°F) mark 4 for 1–1$\frac{1}{2}$ hours until the rice is tender when a few grains are tested.

4 SERVINGS	
kcals	290
kJ	1220
CHO	25 g
Fibre	2 g

VARIATION

BONED AND SKINNED CHICKEN JOINTS can also be given the same treatment. Use fresh or dried tarragon in place of the sage.

Liver Stroganoff

THIS IS AN EXCELLENT METHOD with either lambs', calves' or chickens' livers, as the yogurt tenderises.

INGREDIENTS

450 g (1 lb) calves', lambs' or chickens' liver, sliced into strips

little seasoned flour

60 ml (4 tbsp) oil

2 large onions, skinned and thinly sliced in rings

225 g (8 oz) mushrooms, sliced

salt and freshly ground black pepper or crushed green pepper

300 ml ($\frac{1}{2}$ pint) natural yogurt or half yogurt and half soured cream

15 ml (1 tbsp) finely chopped fresh parsley

pinch of paprika

SERVES 4

■ Roll the liver in the seasoned flour, then shake off any excess. Heat a third of the oil in a non-stick pan and soften the onions, without browning. Lift them out and keep hot. Add another third of the oil and soften the mushrooms but on no account let them become crisp. Return the onions to the pan, mix well and season to taste. Remove the contents of the pan and keep hot. Wipe around the pan with absorbent kitchen paper.

■ Heat the remaining oil and quickly fry the liver strips, turning them over frequently so that they are browned on the outside, while pink within, and making sure that they do not stick together. Put back the onion and mushroom mixture, and stir the liver strips well in.

■ Add the yogurt, or yogurt and soured cream. Mix through lightly and heat through but do not boil or the yogurt will separate. Check for seasoning and adjust if needed. Serve on a warmed dish, sprinkled with parsley and paprika. A purée of potatoes or boiled brown or white rice and a green vegetable make good accompaniments.

4 SERVINGS	
kcals	345
kJ	1445
CHO	10 g
Fibre	3 g

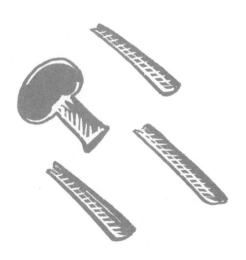

Devilled Kidneys

AN ADMIRABLE LUNCHEON or supper dish. Lamb kidneys are the best for this method. Allow 2–3 kidneys per person.

INGREDIENTS
6 lamb's kidneys, skinned, halved and trimmed
15 ml (1 tbsp) oil
10 ml (2 tsp) Worcestershire sauce
10 ml (2 tsp) mushroom ketchup
100 g (4 oz) butter or margarine
10 ml (2 tsp) dry English mustard powder
freshly ground white pepper
pinch of cayenne pepper
pinch of salt
SERVES 2 – 3

■ Brush the kidney halves with a little oil. Grill them on both sides for about 7 minutes until well browned on the outside but still pink within.

■ Meanwhile, mix all the other ingredients together in a bowl. Just before serving the kidneys, spread the mixture all over them, heat for just 1 minute under the grill and serve at once on a warmed dish.

2 SERVINGS		3 SERVINGS	
kcals	595	kcals	400
kJ	2475	kJ	1650
CHO	Negligible	CHO	Negligible
Fibre	0	Fibre	0

PASTA, RICE AND PULSES

WHOLEWHEAT PASTA IS THE VARIETY that is considered to be best for diabetics, on account of the fibre content. It is essential to have plenty of boiling water to cook pasta of any kind, as this helps to avoid its sticking together. Use about 7 litres (6 quarts) water for every 450 g (1 lb) pasta. The water should first be brought to a good rolling boil and, just before adding the pasta, pour in 15 ml (1 tbsp) sunflower or corn oil, as this also helps to keep the pasta from clumping together. As soon as the water comes back to a vigorous boil, give a good stir to mix it well in the water and to ensure that a strand has not stuck to the bottom of the pot: a wooden Scottish *spirtle*, as used in traditional porridge making, is ideal for this, otherwise use a wooden spoon. Stir, add the salt and maintain an active boiling action: do not let the water sink to a simmer as the turbulence of the water helps both to cook and to keep each piece of pasta separate.

There is an enormous variety of pasta shapes and sizes, and pastas of different compositions have different cooking times. For most dried tagliatelle and spaghetti, the cooking time is about 10–12 minutes, but freshly made pasta may take only 2–5 minutes according to variety. If using the dried pasta, such as spirals or *fusilli*, they need only about 8–10 minutes. All timings should be taken from the time the water returns to the boil after the addition of the pasta. If in doubt, just take out a piece, let it cool and taste it, giving a little more time if you find it too hard. Remember though, while draining in a colander, pasta will continue to soften for a moment or two. Take it out while it has just a tiny trace of firmness left (what the Italians call 'al dente'—to the tooth—if you bite a piece gently, you will see what they mean), then, by the time it has drained, the pasta will be just perfectly cooked.

Pasta must be kept hot while any sauce or flavourings are added. This should be prepared quickly or the pasta can become too soft and mushy. Sauces therefore should always be made ready beforehand and be piping hot, so that they can be mixed in or poured over the pasta right away, then served at once on a warmed dish or individual plates.

Pasta is a perfect food for all occasions; it can be made very simply or, with the addition of more exotic ingredients, it can be transformed into something very special indeed. When, for some years, I lived in Italy, I found many ways of using pasta for delicious meals as it gives true scope for imaginative variation.

Rice is perhaps one of the most resourceful of foods, for it can be used in both sweet and savoury dishes, and also in a variety of invalid foods. It is an annual grass indigenous to India. It was widely cultivated in many countries of the Far East for several millenia B.C. and has become the staple diet of the greatest number of people in the world, chiefly in Asia. Its first large scale cultivation in Europe was near Pisa, Italy, in 1486. Earlier than that, rice is thought to have been introduced into Spain by the Arabs. It was first grown in the New World, in South Carolina, in 1700 and has since then become a very popular food all over the world. Considerably different varieties of rice are used in the different regional cuisines, so the best variety to use in the recipes that follow will be given in each case.

In Italy, rice is to the north what pasta is to the south, and the Piedmontese *arborio* rice is well suited to the slow, long cooking needed to make a good risotto. You will not succeed in making an authentic risotto using a Basmati or other long grained rice. In Italian cuisine, rice is never served as a separate vegetable with poultry, meat or fish; they are always cooked with the rice. There is a single exception, the famous knuckle of veal dish *Ossi Buchi*, see page 81. For this dish, the rice is always cooked and served separately.

Brown rice has a distinct dietetic advantage for diabetics, as it has a better fibre content and should therefore be preferred unless there is a very good reason why a particular dish calls for the white variety.

Pulses, too, are a very important part of the diabetic diet, as they are a good source of fibre, yet low in carbohydrates. They also contain protein and minerals.

The word 'pulses' covers all members of the bean family such as: aduki beans, black beans, black eyed beans, borlotti beans, broad beans, butter beans, cannellini beans, fava beans, field beans, flageolet beans, ful medames, haricot beans, lima beans, mung beans, red kidney beans, soya beans and speckled Mexican beans. It also covers dried peas and split peas, red, green and brown lentils, pigeon peas and chick peas.

As most of the pulses dry well, they are mostly encountered in their dried form, but an increasing number of them are now becoming available in canned or frozen presentations, some of the latter being particularly good. In fact, there is no longer any excuse for remaining with the mushy, tomato sauce soaked variety, which is often sold with sugar added, either in the sauce or in the cooking, so make sure to examine the fine print on the can! Don't forget to check the varieties available in the health food shops and delicatessens as well as in the supermarkets.

You can provide great variety by using different combinations of several kinds of pulses because, as dietary sources, they have a considerable similarity with one another, though the soya bean is different, having a higher protein content.

All dried pulses, with the exception of red lentils, require soaking for some hours before cooking and most require long, slow cooking after a rapid initial boil of 15 minutes. Red kidney beans should never be used unless given that first initial boil as it is needed to destroy a toxin which occurs in the bean itself. However, once boiled rapidly, it is perfectly safe to use them in any quantity.

The time taken to prepare dishes with dried beans can be reduced greatly if you have a pressure cooker, but still soak them in water or stock overnight first. In an emergency, put them into a saucepan, cover with cold water to come above the beans and bring to the boil. Boil for 4 minutes, then remove from the heat and soak for 1 hour. This quick soaking procedure should only be used in a genuine emergency and must be followed by full cooking in the recommended way. The overnight soaking method definitely gives the best results.

In the recipes, the weights of beans given are the weights of the dried beans needed.

Fettucine con Salmone Affumicata—Broad Noodles with Smoked Salmon

A SIMPLE PASTA DISH to prepare with the luxurious touch of smoked salmon.

INGREDIENTS
450 g (1 lb) fettuccini or tagliatelle
30 ml (2 tbsp) olive oil or 25 g (1 oz) butter
100 g (4 oz) smoked salmon or smoked sea trout, chopped into 1 cm (½ inch) pieces
60 ml (4 tbsp) low-fat quark or single cream
squeeze of fresh lemon juice
freshly ground black pepper

SERVES 6 FOR A FIRST COURSE OR 4 FOR A MAIN COURSE

■ Cook the pasta as on page 85. While the pasta is draining, put the rinsed and dried saucepan back on the stove with the oil or butter and heat gently, but do not let it smoke or brown.

▌ Add the drained pasta and turn it gently to coat. Put in the salmon pieces and fold them through the pasta. Stir in the quark. Squeeze in the lemon juice, season with a good grind of black pepper and serve at once on warmed plates.

4 SERVINGS		6 SERVINGS	
kcals	510	kcals	340
kJ	2140	kJ	1425
CHO	75 g	CHO	50 g
Fibre	9 g	Fibre	6 g

VARIATIONS

THIS DISH IS ALSO DELICIOUS using 225 g (8 oz) fresh poached salmon, skinned, boned and flaked, instead of smoked salmon. Use butter in place of oil and add an extra 15 ml (1 tbsp) cream, as well as salt to taste at the end.

Drained flaked canned tuna is also very good prepared this way.

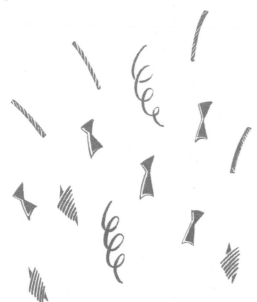

Fusilli con Salsa di Noce—Spirals in Walnut Sauce

THIS DISH IS TRADITIONALLY MADE with spirals, *fusilli*, and the sauce is quite different from any other pasta sauce. It makes a good dish for a first course or for a lunch.

INGREDIENTS
350 g (12 oz) pasta spirals
25 g (1 oz) butter
60 ml (4 tbsp) finely grated Parmesan cheese
For the sauce
20 walnuts, crushed
150 ml ($\frac{1}{4}$ pint) cream
150 g (5 oz) low-fat quark
10 ml (2 tsp) chopped fresh marjoram or 5 ml (1 tsp) dried
salt and freshly ground black pepper
SERVES 6

▌ For the sauce, grind the walnuts in a liquidiser or food processor until reduced to a smooth paste. Blend in the cream and quark. Add the marjoram and seasoning, then blend again for about 1 minute.

▌ Cook the pasta as on page 85. Drain well and mix at once with the butter and Parmesan cheese. Stir the walnut sauce into the pasta, check the seasoning and serve immediately on warmed individual plates.

6 SERVINGS	
kcals	425
kJ	920
CHO	40 g
Fibre	6 g

Risotto Bianco

5 SERVINGS		6 SERVINGS	
kcals	275	kcals	230
kJ	1155	kJ	965
CHO	50 g	CHO	40 g
Fibre	2 g	Fibre	1 g

A LIGHT CHICKEN or vegetable stock is best for this rich dish.

INGREDIENTS

25 g (1 oz) butter
1 small onion, skinned and finely chopped
275 g (10 oz) arborio rice
150 ml (¼ pint) dry white wine
1 litre (1¾ pints) stock or water
knob of butter to serve
30 ml (2 tbsp) finely grated Parmesan cheese

SERVES 5 – 6

▮ Melt the butter in a heavy deep pan or metal casserole and lightly fry the onion until soft and golden. Add the rice and stir well until every grain has been coated, but do not brown. Add the wine and cook over a medium heat until the wine has almost completely been absorbed.

▮ Add the stock, a cupful at a time, stirring each one in. Add the next cupful of stock when the previous one has almost been absorbed. When the last cupful has been added, cook very gently on the top of the stove, uncovered, for 20 minutes, **without stirring**.

▮ Test a few grains of rice between the fingers, if the grains are still firm and all the liquid is absorbed, add about 45 ml (3 tbsp) water and stir gently with a wooden fork. Test again when the liquid has been absorbed, but be careful not to let the rice become mushy by overcooking. Serve at once with a knob of butter and Parmesan cheese.

VARIATIONS

FOR RISOTTO MILANESE, add 30–40 ml (2–3 tbsp) raw beef marrow chunks to the butter before cooking the rice. When the stock is being added, gently stir in a few strands of saffron with the stock. Finally just before serving, lightly fork in 15 g (½ oz) butter, in little pieces, and the same amount of finely grated Parmesan cheese using a wooden fork.

For RISOTTO CON FUNGHI, or with shellfish, add 225 g (8 oz) chopped mushrooms, or chopped shrimps or prawns after the wine, but leave out the beef marrow.

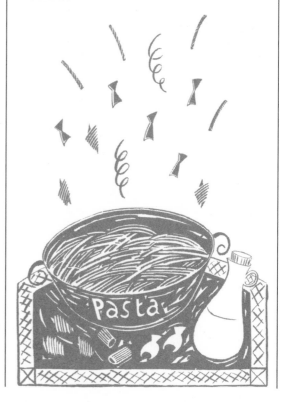

Pasta Giorgio

THIS IS A VERY fresh-tasting pasta dish which is easy to make.

INGREDIENTS

350 g (12 oz) pasta spirals or tagliatelle
30 ml (2 tbsp) olive oil
salt
1 large red pepper, cored, deseeded and chopped
2 garlic cloves, skinned and chopped
2 large ripe tomatoes, skinned and coarsely chopped
25 g (1 oz) pinenut kernels
12 black olives, stoned and chopped
15 ml (1 tbsp) chopped fresh basil leaves or 5 ml (1 tsp) dried
freshly ground black pepper
Parmesan cheese, finely grated, to serve

SERVES 4 – 6

▪ Cook the pasta as on page 85. While the pasta is draining, put the rinsed and dried saucepan back on the stove with the olive oil and soften the pepper and garlic. Add the tomatoes and soften thoroughly, mixing well.

▪ Gently fold in the drained pasta, then add the pinenut kernels, olives, basil and give a good grind of black pepper. Serve at once on warmed plates, accompanied by Parmesan cheese.

4 SERVINGS		6 SERVINGS	
kcals	425	kcals	285
kJ	1780	kJ	1190
CHO	60 g	CHO	40 g
Fibre	9 g	Fibre	6 g

Pasta con le Zucchine

THIS IS A SOUTHERN ITALIAN DISH, simple and delicious. In Italy, it is usually considered too delicately flavoured a dish to eat with Parmesan, but this is a matter of individual choice.

INGREDIENTS

450 g (1 lb) pasta of your choice
60 ml (4 tbsp) olive oil or 50 g (2 oz) butter
450 g (1 lb) courgettes, unpeeled, thinly sliced
salt and freshly ground black pepper
30 ml (2 tbsp) cream or low-fat quark

SERVES 4 – 6

▪ Cook the pasta as on page 85. While cooking, heat the oil or butter (or a mixture of the two if you prefer) and lightly fry the courgettes until soft, but do not allow them to brown. Set aside and keep hot.

▪ Drain the pasta and return it to the rinsed and drained saucepan over a very low heat. Gently fold in the courgettes and oil or butter. Season to taste. Finally, gently mix in the cream or quark and serve at once.

4 SERVINGS		6 SERVINGS	
kcals	445	kcals	295
kJ	1860	kJ	1245
CHO	60 g	CHO	40 g
Fibre	7 g	Fibre	5 g

VARIATION

INSTEAD OF THE COURGETTES, use slices of peeled, stoned avocado and lightly cook in a little butter. Fold into the drained pasta and scatter with finely grated Parmesan cheese.

Spanish Rice

4 SERVINGS	
kcals	240
kJ	1010
CHO	35 g
Fibre	5 g

A VERY FILLING DISH, as it uses beans as well as rice. Served cold, it makes an excellent salad.

INGREDIENTS
15 ml (1 tbsp) oil
1 large Spanish onion, skinned and finely chopped
1 garlic clove, skinned and crushed
4 large ripe tomatoes, skinned and chopped
60 ml (4 tbsp) finely chopped fresh parsley
5 ml (1 tsp) finely chopped fresh marjoram or 2.5 ml ($\frac{1}{2}$ tsp) dried
30 ml (2 tbsp) stock
salt and freshly ground black pepper
225 g (8 oz) long grain brown rice, cooked, cold
225 g (8 oz) red kidney beans, canned without added sugar, drained
To garnish
12 black olives, stoned and halved
2 hard-boiled eggs, size 3, quartered
10 ml (2 tsp) chopped fresh chives
10 ml (2 tsp) chopped fresh parsley
SERVES 4

■ Heat the oil in a flameproof casserole on the top of the stove and cook the onion until soft but not coloured. Add the garlic, tomatoes and herbs and soften them, then add the stock. Bring to the boil, season, cover and cook very gently for 10 minutes, stirring occasionally to make sure that there is no sticking.

■ Put in the rice and beans, mix thoroughly with a wooden fork and heat through. Transfer to a warmed serving dish and garnish with the olives, eggs, chives and parsley.

Oriental Rice

A DELIGHTFUL RICE DISH which can be eaten hot or cold.

INGREDIENTS
200 g (7 oz) long grain brown rice, washed and drained
2 shallots or small onions, skinned and finely chopped
1 garlic clove, skinned and crushed
5 ml (1 tsp) ground coriander
2.5 ml ($\frac{1}{2}$ tsp) ground cumin
1.25 ml ($\frac{1}{4}$ tsp) ground chilli
5 ml (1 tsp) salt (omit if a cube has been used to make stock)
freshly ground black pepper
750 ml (1$\frac{1}{4}$ pints) chicken stock
175 g (6 oz) bean sprouts, drained if canned
100 g (4 oz) shrimps, peeled, drained if canned
1 egg, size 3, beaten
SERVES 4

■ Put the rice, shallots, garlic, spices and seasoning into an ovenproof casserole and pour over the stock. Cover and bake at 180°C (350°F) mark 4 for 1 hour. Stir in the bean sprouts and shrimps, cover again and return to the oven for a further 15 minutes.

■ Meanwhile, beat the egg in a bowl with 15 ml (1 tbsp) cold water and pour over the base of a non-stick pan over a low heat. When the egg has set on the bottom, cut into strips about 1 cm ($\frac{1}{2}$ inch) wide. Turn them over with a slice, then remove from the heat and keep warm.

■ Check the rice has absorbed all the liquid, if not, cook for a further 5 minutes or so. Fluff up with a wooden fork, lay the egg strips lattice-wise across the top and serve at once.

4 SERVINGS	
kcals	240
kJ	1015
CHO	45 g
Fibre	2 g

VARIATIONS

COOKED CHICKEN OR HAM, finely chopped, can be used instead of shrimps.

The dish can be made in a vegetarian way, using quarters of hard-boiled eggs, omitting the egg strips.

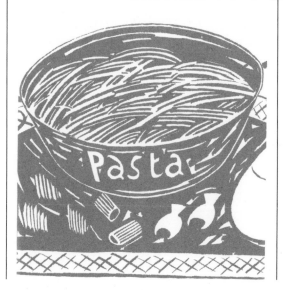

Brown Rice Pilaff

THIS PILAFF IS DELICIOUS served with lentils, vegetables or with a casserole dish, particularly vegetarian.

INGREDIENTS
30 ml (2 tbsp) vegetable oil
3 medium onions, skinned and finely chopped
1 large red pepper, cored, deseeded and chopped
1 large garlic clove, skinned and crushed
5 ml (1 tsp) ground turmeric
225 g (8 oz) long grain brown rice
900 ml (1½ pints) vegetable stock
15 ml (1 tbsp) freshly squeezed lemon juice or white wine vinegar
salt and freshly ground black pepper
SERVES 4

■ Heat the oil in a flameproof casserole and lightly fry the onions and pepper until soft but not browned. Add the garlic and turmeric, stirring well. Add the rice, continuing to stir, so that it is well coated with the oil and spice. Pour in the stock and lemon juice. Season to taste. Bring to the boil and cover.

■ Bake at 180°C (350°F) mark 4 for about 1¼ hours until all the liquid is absorbed. Lightly fork through with a wooden fork to make the rice fluffy before serving.

4 SERVINGS	
kcals	275
kJ	1170
CHO	50 g
Fibre	3 g

COOKING DRIED BEANS AND OTHER DRIED PULSES

SOAK THE BEANS IN UNSALTED WATER overnight. Drain, then put into a pan large enough to take the beans and sufficient water or stock to give a depth of 2.5 cm (1 inch) above the beans and allow enough space for boiling up. Bring to the boil and boil rapidly for 15 minutes, then lower the heat to a gentle simmer. At this point it is a good idea to add a large onion, skinned and sliced, and a sprig of thyme for every 225 g (8 oz) beans. **Do not salt** at this stage, but leave until the beans are cooked or you will make them hard. Partially cover the pan and maintain at a low simmer for $1-1\frac{1}{2}$ hours or until the beans are soft but not mushy. Leave in their liquid in a cool place until required. Drain them, reserving the liquid which makes an excellent vegetable stock for soups and stews of many kinds.

Chick peas need far longer cooking, at least 2 hours should be allowed before testing. Remember too that long cooking may result in the beans or chick peas becoming dry and sticking to the bottom of the pan, so check them occasionally and add a little stock or water if needed and a gentle stir. Lentils are particularly prone to drying out if cooked in an aluminium saucepan with a thin bottom and so are best cooked in a heavy cast iron pot.

PRESSURE COOKING PULSES

HERE ARE PRESSURE COOKING TIMES at full pressure:

Aduki, field and mung beans, peas, split peas and red lentils will take 12–15 minutes.

Black-eyed, black, borlotti, cannellini, ful medames, lima beans and green and brown lentils will take 25 minutes.

Broad, butter, haricot, speckled Mexican and red kidney beans will take about 45 minutes.

Chick peas and soya beans will take as much as $1-1\frac{1}{2}$ hours at full pressure.

It is a good plan to cook a large number of pulses at a time, both for convenience and economy as once cooked they will keep for about 4 days in the refrigerator and for about 2 months in the freezer.

One last point to note, in cooking, salt and any acid ingredients such as tomato, tomato juice or lemon juice should never be added until the beans are completely cooked and soft, as they will have the effect of making the beans permanently hard.

Because it is efficient and economical to cook the pulses in large batches, you are likely to have some leftovers. There are such a great variety of delicious salads, soups, quick meals and additions to other dishes that can use them up, for example, see Spanish rice on page 90. In Tuscany, a salad of haricot beans is invariably served with grilled steak and other roast meats.

Cassoulet

THE TRUE FRENCH CASSOULET is a great deal more complicated than this version and contains other meats, including some preserved goose. However, this simplified version of beans baked with bacon can be very acceptable on a cold winter's day.

INGREDIENTS

225 g (8 oz) haricot beans, soaked overnight
15 ml (1 tbsp) olive oil
1 medium onion, skinned and sliced
2 garlic cloves, skinned and crushed
2.5 ml ($\frac{1}{2}$ tsp) chopped fresh thyme
2.5 ml ($\frac{1}{2}$ tsp) dried marjoram
450 g (1 lb) piece lean collar bacon, soaked
1 medium onion, skinned and stuck with 2 whole cloves
10 ml (2 tsp) tomato purée
2 medium or large ripe tomatoes, skinned and coarsely chopped
100 g (4 oz) garlic salami or garlic sausage, derinded and chopped
salt and freshly ground black pepper

SERVES 4

■ Drain the beans, put them into a medium saucepan and cover with cold water to come 2.5 cm (1 inch) over the beans. Bring to the boil and simmer gently for 40 minutes. Drain and put them into a large flameproof casserole.

■ Heat the oil in a pan and soften the sliced onion, then add it to the beans together with the garlic and the herbs. Mix and set aside, covered.

■ Throw away the bacon soaking water and cover with fresh cold water. Bring to the boil, add the onion stuck with cloves and simmer for about 30 minutes. Lift out the bacon, peel off and discard the skin. Cut the bacon into large pieces and mix with the beans and onion.

■ Taste the bacon stock and, if it is not too salty, measure out 450 ml ($\frac{3}{4}$ pint), if too salty use the same amount of water. Warm the stock or water, add and dissolve the tomato purée. Add the tomatoes, then pour the mixture over the beans and bacon, barely covering, but reserve any remaining stock.

■ Cover and braise at 170°C (325°F) mark 3 for about 45 minutes to 1 hour. Take out and test one of the beans for tenderness, if soft, add the garlic salami or sausage chunks and mix them well in. If the beans are becoming too dry, add a little more stock or water. Taste for seasoning, being cautious with salt, but add plenty of freshly ground black pepper. Cook, uncovered, for a further 20–25 minutes. Serve from the casserole, accompanied by crusty, hot fresh bread and a green salad.

4 SERVINGS	
kcals	535
kJ	2245
CHO	30 g
Fibre	15 g

VARIATION

LEFTOVER JOINTS OF POULTRY or game can be added.

Hummus

AN EXCELLENT SPREAD from the Eastern Mediterranean which makes a stimulating first course or even a part of a mixed salad for a main meal. Spread on small water biscuits, hummus also makes an excellent accompaniment to drinks. If you are fond of garlic, you can increase the quantity to your taste. A word about the sesame seeds; the best for this dish are the dehusked variety: to toast them simply put into a large heavy, absolutely dry, hot pan and toast until golden, which they do very quickly. Take them out before they brown.

INGREDIENTS

225 g (8 oz) chick peas, cooked (see page 92), or canned, without added sugar, drained

60 ml (4 tbsp) sesame seeds, dehusked and freshly toasted

2 large garlic cloves, skinned and crushed with a pinch of sea salt

30 ml (2 tbsp) freshly squeezed lemon juice

pinch of ground cumin

45 ml (3 tbsp) olive oil

salt and freshly ground black pepper

30 ml (2 tbsp) finely chopped fresh parsley

SERVES 6 – 8

■ Process the chick peas until smooth in a food processor or liquidiser, or sieve them.
■ Put three-quarters of the sesame seeds into a mortar and pound into a paste. Blend the paste well into the chick pea purée. Reserve the remaining toasted sesame seeds for garnishing.
■ Blend in the garlic, then the lemon juice and finally the cumin, making sure that each is evenly mixed before adding the next. Alternatively, beat them into the purée with a wooden spoon. Gradually add the oil. When the purée is quite smooth, taste for seasoning and correct to your taste. Finally, add half the parsley, keeping the rest for garnishing.
■ Press the hummus into a cold bowl and chill. To serve, turn out on to a serving dish, scatter over the remaining toasted sesame seeds and parsley. Accompany with wholemeal bread or rolls.

6 SERVINGS		8 SERVINGS	
kcals	150	kcals	115
kJ	635	kJ	475
CHO	10 g	CHO	5 g
Fibre	3 g	Fibre	2 g

Bean and Celery Pâté

AN EASILY MADE, deliciously smooth yet crunchy pâté.

INGREDIENTS

100 g (4 oz) cooked butter beans, drained if canned

30 ml (2 tbsp) olive oil

1 small onion, skinned and finely chopped

1 garlic clove, skinned and finely chopped

1 celery heart, trimmed and finely chopped

30 ml (2 tbsp) crunchy peanut butter

15 ml (1 tbsp) cider vinegar

salt and freshly ground black pepper or crushed green pepper

10 ml (2 tsp) finely chopped fresh parsley, to garnish

SERVES 4

■ Put the beans in a liquidiser or food processor and process for $\frac{1}{2}$ minute.

Alternatively, put them through a mouli legume or rub through a sieve.

▌ Heat the oil in a pan and soften the onion, garlic and celery, without letting them brown. Add to the beans with any remaining oil, the peanut butter and cider vinegar. Season to taste. Process for another minute on HIGH, or beat the mixture into the sieved beans with a wooden spoon.

▌ Turn out the pâté on to a serving dish and mound up. Chill in the refrigerator until firm. Just before serving, scatter with the finely chopped parsley. Serve with toast.

4 SERVINGS	
kcals	130
kJ	545
CHO	5 g
Fibre	3 g

VARIATIONS

A MEDIUM COOKING APPLE, peeled, cored and chopped, can be used in place of celery.

Almost any other variety of cooked pulses can be substituted for the butter beans.

Hazelnut or walnut butter (easily made in the food processor) can be used in place of the peanut butter.

Lenticchie del Primo d'Anno—New Year's Day Lentils

IN ITALY, it is thought that to eat this on New Year's Day will bring good fortune!

INGREDIENTS
30 ml (2 tbsp) finely chopped fresh parsley
2 celery stalks, trimmed and finely chopped
1 garlic clove, skinned and chopped
1 medium onion, skinned and chopped
2 slices of salt pork or bacon, derinded and finely chopped
30 ml (2 tbsp) olive oil
15 ml (1 tbsp) tomato purée
225 g (8 oz) brown or green lentils, soaked overnight and drained
750 ml (1½ pints) hot stock or water
SERVES 4

▌ Mix the parsley, celery, garlic, onion and salt pork or bacon well together. Heat the oil in a large, heavy-based saucepan and sauté the mixture until golden. Mix the tomato purée well in. Add the drained lentils and mix thoroughly.

▌ Pour in the hot stock or water, mix well and bring to the boil. Simmer, covered, for about 1 hour, stirring from time to time and checking that the bottom does not catch. Test a few lentils to see if they are soft and, if not, cook a little longer. Season and serve with Italian garlic sausage.

4 SERVINGS	
kcals	255
kJ	1070
CHO	30 g
Fibre	8 g

SALADS AND VEGETABLES

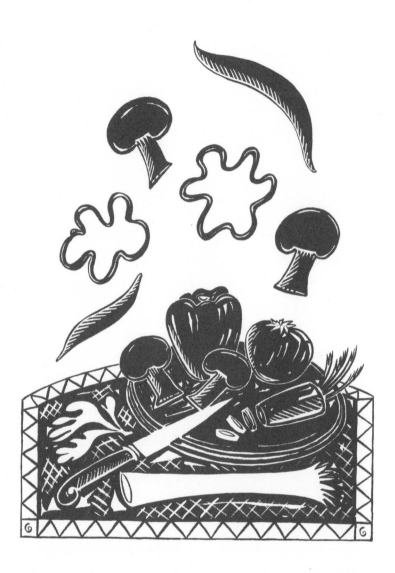

WHEN THE REALLY HOT WEATHER comes, salads attain their greatest appeal, and the light but filling salad has recently grown in popularity. They are so adaptable, for their composition can be so greatly varied. You can also serve salads as a main course, with poultry, ham, fish, eggs or cheese. There are many good economical, yet nutritious, combinations that can give a balanced food and fibre intake most suitable for diabetics. Particularly when we remember that a sedentary occupation in a centrally heated office or factory poses dietetic problems for many people.

Vegetables should be treated with the respect that they deserve and always cooked in ways that will preserve their nutritive values, their delicious flavours and their great variety of texture. They have many important properties necessary in our daily diet, especially to those of us who are diabetics, where a high fibre

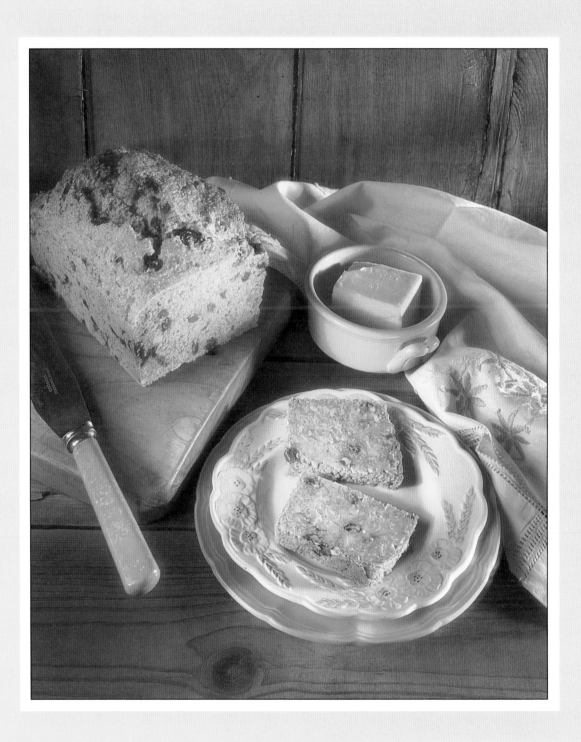

Irish Farmhouse Loaf (page 121)

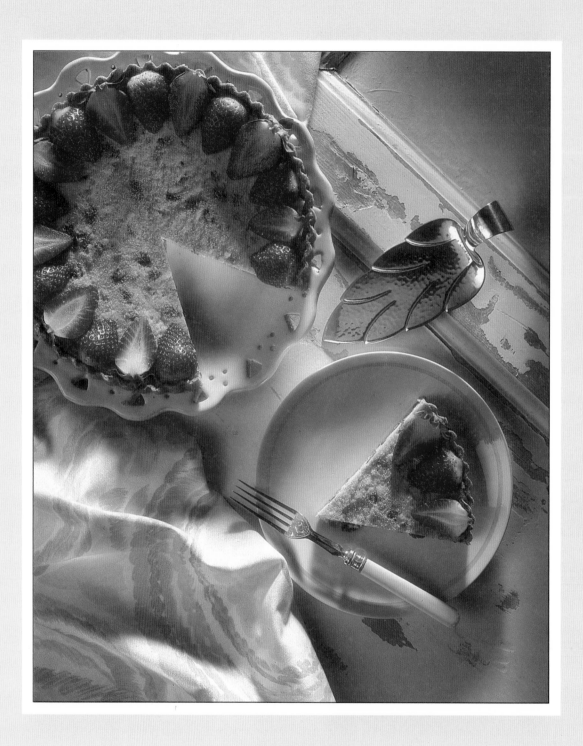

Curd Tart (page 132)

intake helps. Vegetables should never be abused in cooking, a widespread practice, by being boiled for far too long in an excess of water, which is then tipped away carrying with it most of the minerals and vitamins. The sad-looking vegetables left behind are virtually devoid of any nutritive value and even the fibre has been so broken down as to be almost useless.

We should realise that vegetables are not always to be relegated to an accompanying role. There are many that can, properly treated, make an excellent main course in themselves, with the addition of a little cheese, eggs or a small quantity of meat or fish and, of course, the use of an appropriate and attractive sauce. Some of the more exotic vegetables now available to many of us are expensive, but remember that there should be very little waste on good clean vegetables, and also that an occasional change in our food is one of the best and healthiest tonics that we can take.

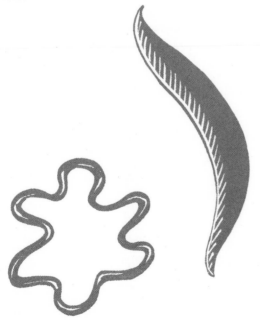

Greek Country Salad

AN EXTREMELY GOOD FIRST COURSE or light main meal, best made with Feta cheese.

INGREDIENTS
1 crisp lettuce, preferably cos or iceberg
1 red pepper, cored, deseeded and finely sliced
2 small onions or shallots, skinned and sliced
3 large tomatoes, skinned and sliced
1 garlic clove, skinned and sliced
$\frac{1}{2}$ medium cucumber, peeled and sliced
salt and freshly ground black pepper
100–150 g (4–5 oz) Feta cheese or Caerphilly, diced
50 g (2 oz) black olives, stoned, to garnish (optional)
For the dressing
30 ml (2 tbsp) freshly squeezed lemon juice
45–60 ml (3–4 tbsp) olive oil
SERVES 4

■ Line a salad bowl with the lettuce leaves. Arrange the pepper, onions, tomatoes, garlic and cucumber in layers, seasoning each layer. Be sparing with the salt if using Feta cheese as it can be salty. Put the diced cheese on top and add more pepper.

■ Mix the dressing ingredients together vigorously. Pour over the salad and scatter the olives on top, if using. If you wish, instead of using a salad bowl, this salad can be made up on individual plates, but they need to be capacious and fairly deep.

4 SERVINGS	
kcals	240
kJ	1000
CHO	5 g
Fibre	3 g

Waldorf Salad

A CRUNCHY FAVOURITE OF MINE which is delicious with a full fat soft cheese or quark, hard-boiled eggs, tuna fish or poultry.

INGREDIENTS

450 g (1 lb) red, crisp eating apples, cored but unpeeled
freshly squeezed juice of $\frac{1}{2}$ lemon
1 crisp cos lettuce, thinly sliced
2 crisp celery hearts, trimmed and thinly sliced
50 g (2 oz) walnuts, chopped into quarters
For the dressing
25 ml (1$\frac{1}{2}$ tbsp) olive or walnut oil
10 ml (2 tsp) cider vinegar
salt and freshly ground black pepper

SERVES 4 AS A SIDE SALAD

■ Slice the apples across fairly thickly, then halve the slices and dice them. Sprinkle well with the lemon juice to avoid them becoming brown. Put the apple in a bowl, pour over the remaining lemon juice and leave for about 15 minutes.

■ Mix well together the apples, lettuce, celery and walnuts in a bowl.

■ Shake the dressing ingredients well together in a screw-topped jar. Season to taste. About 20 minutes before serving, give the dressing another good shake, pour it over the salad, mix well and transfer to a serving dish.

4 SERVINGS	
kcals	160
kJ	670
CHO	15 g
Fibre	5 g

Carrot and Apple Salad

THIS IS PARTICULARLY REFRESHING and delicious when served with a portion of curd cheese or quark, into which some fresh herbs have been mixed.

INGREDIENTS

225 g (8 oz) young carrots, scraped and coarsely grated
4 small eating apples, peeled and grated, preferably Cox's Orange Pippins
freshly squeezed juice of 1 lemon
salt

SERVES 2 – 3

■ Mix the grated carrots and apples together in a bowl.

■ Pour over the lemon juice, add a little salt and mix well. Taste to ensure that there is enough salt, correct if necessary and leave for 1 hour to marinate.

2 SERVINGS		3 SERVINGS	
kcals	95	kcals	65
kJ	410	kJ	270
CHO	25 g	CHO	15 g
Fibre	6 g	Fibre	4 g

VARIATION

ABOUT 30–40 ml (2–3 tbsp) sultanas can also be added before the lemon juice is poured over.

Mushoshi

AN ARMENIAN LENTIL SALAD with a captivating and unusual taste. Good with cheese or hard-boiled eggs.

INGREDIENTS

100 g (4 oz) brown lentils, rinsed
salt
1 small onion, skinned and chopped
75 g (3 oz) dried apricots, soaked and chopped
50 g (2 oz) walnuts, chopped
30 ml (2 tbsp) chopped fresh parsley
For the dressing
30 ml (2 tbsp) olive oil
25 ml (1½ tbsp) freshly squeezed lemon juice
salt and freshly ground black pepper

SERVES 3 – 4

▪ Cook the lentils (as on page 92), but do not let them become mushy. Add salt to taste. Stir in the onion, apricots and walnuts and cook for a further 15 minutes. Drain, reserving the liquid for stock, and leave to cool. Put into a deep serving bowl.

▪ Shake together the ingredients for the dressing in a screw-topped jar. Pour over the lentil mixture and mix well in. Scatter the parsley over and serve.

3 SERVINGS		4 SERVINGS	
kcals	310	kcals	235
kJ	1305	kJ	980
CHO	30 g	CHO	25 g
Fibre	12 g	Fibre	9 g

VARIATION

MANY DIFFERENT KINDS OF BEANS can be used instead of lentils.

Salad Elena

AN INVENTION OF MY GRANDMOTHER'S, who named it after a friend of hers. It is exquisite with cold salmon or poultry and looks most attractive.

INGREDIENTS

225 g (8 oz) strawberries, hulled
1 small cucumber, peeled
salt and freshly ground black pepper
30 ml (2 tbsp) dry white wine

SERVES 4 AS AN ACCOMPANIMENT

▪ Slice the strawberries, not too thinly, reserving one whole. Slice the cucumber fairly thinly. Arrange a circle of strawberries around the outside of a large round plate, then add a circle of cucumber, slightly overlapping, inside that and so on alternately until the centre is reached. Put an unsliced strawberry in the middle.

▪ Sprinkle a tiny quantity of freshly ground black pepper on the strawberries, which brings out their flavour, and a very little salt on to the cucumber. Cover and leave in a cool place for 30 minutes.

▪ To serve, very gently dribble the white wine over the salad, but do not make the salad too moist. Serve at once.

4 SERVINGS	
kcals	25
kJ	100
CHO	5 g
Fibre	1 g

Peperonata

A VERSATILE ITALIAN DISH which can be a first course, an omelette filling or an accompaniment to hot or cold meats.

INGREDIENTS

15 ml (1 tbsp) olive oil
15 g (½ oz) butter
1 large onion, skinned and finely sliced
4 peppers, cored, deseeded and sliced
salt and freshly ground black pepper
6 ripe tomatoes, skinned and chopped, or 425 g (15 oz) can tomatoes, drained
2 garlic cloves, skinned and sliced

SERVES 4

■ Heat the oil and butter in a pan and cook the onion until soft but not brown. Add the pepper, season to taste and soften for 15 minutes on a very low heat with the pan covered.

■ When the onions and peppers are soft, add the tomatoes and garlic, season again, mix well and cook very gently in the covered pan for another 30 minutes.

4 SERVINGS	
kcals	95
kJ	395
CHO	10 g
Fibre	3 g

VARIATION

WHEN THE PEPERONATA IS COOKED, oil an ovenproof dish and add the peperonata. Beat 2 eggs and mix them in thoroughly. Bake at 200°C (400°F) mark 6 for 20 minutes. This dish resembles a French pipérade. Served with toast, it makes an excellent first course.

Tabbouleh

THIS LEBANESE RECIPE makes an excellent first course, or it can be served as an accompaniment for a buffet. Tabbouleh uses a lot of fresh herbs, so it is really a dish not to be attempted before late in the spring, nor too late in the autumn. Burghul (cracked wheat) can be bought today at most health food shops. Select the finely ground variety.

INGREDIENTS

50 g (2 oz) burghul (cracked wheat), finely ground and soaked
salt and freshly ground black pepper
freshly squeezed juice of 2 lemons
90 ml (6 tbsp) olive oil
100 g (4 oz) fresh flat leaved parsley, finely chopped
50 g (2 oz) fresh mint, finely chopped
200 g (7 oz) spring onions, trimmed and finely chopped, or 1 large sweet Spanish onion, skinned and finely chopped
To garnish
young crisp cos or iceberg lettuce leaves
3 medium tomatoes, skinned and diced

SERVES 4

■ Soak the burghul for 10 minutes in water to cover. Drain and squeeze or press to remove the excess water. Put it into a large bowl, season to taste, add the juice of 1 lemon and 45 ml (3 tbsp) oil. Mix well and leave to soak for 30–40 minutes.

■ Meanwhile, prepare the herbs. Remove the stalks as only the leaves should be used. Chop them very finely. If using a food processor, be sure you do not process too long and produce a mushy mixture. It is really safer to chop them finely on a chopping board with a sharp knife.

▪ After the burghul has absorbed the first amount of lemon juice and oil, add some of the chopped herbs, enough to give a green, speckled effect, and mix well in. Add the spring onions, more of the lemon juice and oil to taste, then check the seasoning, adjusting if needed. The lemon juice should dominate the oil and the salad should be quite sharp in flavour.

▪ Serve on a large flat serving dish or on individual ones, surrounded by the crisp lettuce leaves (which the Lebanese use as scoops). Top with the tomatoes and any remaining chopped herbs and dressing. Accompany with hot pitta bread.

4 SERVINGS	
kcals	240
kJ	990
CHO	15 g
Fibre	6 g

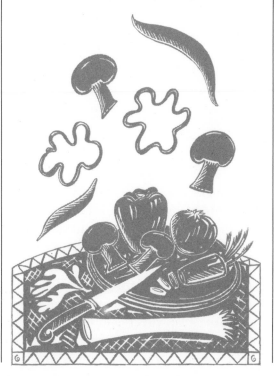

Red Cabbage with Apple

RED CABBAGE IS EXCEEDINGLY GOOD served with game, especially venison, and all kinds of pork and goulash-type dishes. It should be cooked slowly for several hours. This dish freezes well after cooking and is an unusual vegetable in that it improves by long cooking. It can be served cold and also reheats successfully.

INGREDIENTS
15 g (½ oz) butter or margarine
1 large onion, skinned and sliced
1 large cooking apple, peeled, cored and sliced
1 medium red cabbage, trimmed and finely shredded
300 ml (½ pint) stock
4 whole cloves
4 allspice berries or pinch of ground allspice
15–30 ml (1–2 tbsp) red wine or red wine vinegar
salt and freshly ground black pepper
SERVES 8

▪ Heat the butter in a pan and just soften the onion and apple. Add the cabbage, stock, spices, wine and seasoning.

▪ Bring to the boil and simmer gently for about 2 hours or until the cabbage is quite soft. Taste again for seasoning before serving and correct if necessary.

8 SERVINGS	
kcals	45
kJ	185
CHO	5 g
Fibre	3 g

Mollie's Brown Rice Salad

THIS IS ONE OF the most delightful rice salads, given to me by a good friend. It is essential that the peppers, raisins and nuts are very finely chopped.

INGREDIENTS

225 g (8 oz) long grain brown rice, cooked and drained (see page 85)

1 medium red pepper, cored, deseeded and very finely chopped

50 g (2 oz) raisins, very finely chopped

50 g (2 oz) cashew nuts, very finely chopped

30 ml (2 tbsp) chopped spring onions, onion tops or chives

For the dressing

45 ml (3 tbsp) olive oil

30 ml (2 tbsp) soy sauce

30 ml (2 tbsp) freshly squeezed lemon juice

1 garlic clove, skinned and finely chopped

5 ml (1 tsp) peeled and finely chopped fresh root ginger

salt and freshly ground black pepper

30 ml (2 tbsp) finely chopped fresh parsley

SERVES 6 – 8

■ In a large bowl, mix the rice, pepper, raisins, cashew nuts and spring onions.

■ Mix together the ingredients for the dressing, either beating with a fork or shaking hard in a screw-topped jar. Pour over the salad, mix well and serve the rice salad at once.

6 SERVINGS		8 SERVINGS	
kcals	175	kcals	130
kJ	730	kJ	540
CHO	20 g	CHO	15 g
Fibre	2 g	Fibre	1 g

Stuffed Vegetables

STUFFED VEGETABLES MAKE ONE of the most economical yet satisfying meals, and this particularly applies to marrows, courgettes, peppers, aubergines, large onions and cabbage, spinach or vine leaves. Either fresh or cooked meat can be used, but pork should always be cooked first.

The following stuffing ingredients will be enough for 1 medium marrow, 8 courgettes, 4 medium peppers, 2 medium aubergines or 6–8 medium cabbage, spinach or vine leaves.

INGREDIENTS

450 ml (¾ pint) stock or 15 ml (1 tbsp) tomato purée in 450 ml (¾ pint) hot water

25–30 ml (1½–2 tbsp) grated cheese

For the stuffing

225 g (8 oz) minced cooked beef, lamb, pork or chicken, or for vegetarians, mushrooms, tomatoes, beans and chopped nuts

60 ml (4 tbsp) cooked brown rice or cooked pasta, chopped

5 ml (1 tsp) dried marjoram or tarragon

1 garlic clove, skinned and chopped

salt and freshly ground black pepper

1 egg, size 4, beaten

SERVES ABOUT 4

■ To make the stuffing, mix all the stuffing ingredients together, adding the egg last. If the mixture seems too dry, add 15 ml (1 tbsp) of the stock. Set aside.

■ Marrows should be peeled but courgettes should have their skins left on, both should be cut in half lengthwise and deseeded. Cut aubergines in the same way, scatter a little salt on them and leave for 30 minutes. The flesh should then be

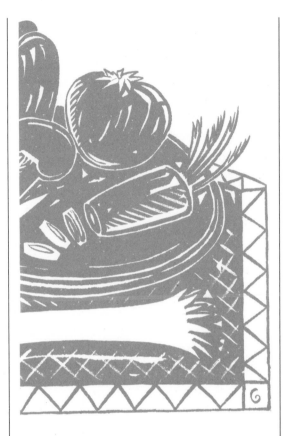

15–20 minutes. If liked, the chopped centre of the courgettes or aubergines can be softened in a little hot oil in the pan and mixed with the stuffing ingredients. Do not allow the vegetable cases to get too soft and floppy, as they must retain their firmness to hold together when they are stuffed and during the final baking. Drain them thoroughly, then pat dry with absorbent kitchen paper before stuffing.

■ Fill the vegetable cases with the stuffing to come at least 1 cm ($\frac{1}{3}$ inch) over the top of the vegetable case, as it will shrink in cooking. Arrange the stuffed vegetables, open end up, side by side in an ovenproof dish, making sure that the size of the dish will allow the vegetable cases to support one another without room for them to fall over. Fold cabbage, spinach and vine leaves around a ball of the stuffing mixture. Place in the dish with the fold downwards to hold it closed. Pack together in the dish to stop them unwrapping.

■ Pour the stock or diluted tomato purée around to a depth of 3 cm (1$\frac{1}{4}$ inches), then top each case with cheese. Cover with a lid or lightly with foil. Cook at 190°C (375°F) mark 5 for 35–45 minutes.

4 SERVINGS	
kcals	190
kJ	790
CHO	5 g
Fibre	0

VARIATION

THE COURGETTES, aubergines or peppers are also excellent served cold, but not chilled.

NOTE: The vegetables to be stuffed will add relatively few kcals, kJ and CHO.

carefully scooped out of the centre, leaving the shell with about 1 cm ($\frac{1}{3}$ inch) flesh evenly around inside the skin. If the flesh is not too seedy, chop and reserve. Cut peppers around the stalk with a sharp knife and remove the core with its seeds. Any seeds that may have fallen into the interior can be scooped out with a long handled spoon. Select unblemished cabbage and spinach leaves, and remove the hard part of the stalk at the base. Steam the leaves over boiling water for about 3 minutes to blanch them. Vine leaves need only to be blanched. Marrows, courgettes and peppers should also be steamed, before stuffing—4 minutes for marrow, 3 minutes for courgette or pepper. Brush aubergines with oil. Bake at 180°C (350°F) mark 4 for about

Stir-Fried Vegetables

A SIMPLE AND QUICK WAY of cooking many kinds of vegetables that preserves the nutrients, flavours and textures. The choice of vegetables used is a matter of preference. The thin slicing of the vegetables is one of the keys to success and any tough or dried parts should be discarded. A wok is ideal, but a large, heavy frying pan is also good. I like the following mixture.

INGREDIENTS
45 ml (3 tbsp) oil
1 head of celery, trimmed and thinly sliced
2 medium peppers, cored, deseeded and thinly sliced
1 small onion, skinned and thinly sliced
150 g (5 oz) mushrooms, thinly sliced
$\frac{1}{2}$ head of white cabbage, trimmed and thinly shredded
15 ml (1 tbsp) soy sauce or to taste
50–75 g (2–3 oz) bean sprouts or sliced bamboo shoots (optional)
SERVES 4 – 5

■ Heat a wok or large frying pan and add 15 ml (1 tbsp) of the oil. When the oil is hot, add the celery and peppers and cook quickly, shaking the wok or pan and stirring constantly. Do not allow the vegetables to take colour and lower the heat if necessary.

■ When soft, add the onion and soften, adding a little more oil if needed and mixing all the vegetables together as they cook. Add the remaining oil, the mushrooms, then the cabbage. Finally add the soy sauce to taste.

■ The complete cooking time should not take more than about 7 minutes or until all the vegetables, though softened, are still crunchy. If using bean sprouts or bamboo shoots, these should go in after the cabbage but before the soy sauce. If from a can, drain first. Accompany with boiled brown rice and serve immediately as this is not a dish that can be kept waiting.

4 SERVINGS		5 SERVINGS	
kcals	115	kcals	95
kJ	485	kJ	390
CHO	5 g	CHO	5 g
Fibre	4 g	Fibre	3 g

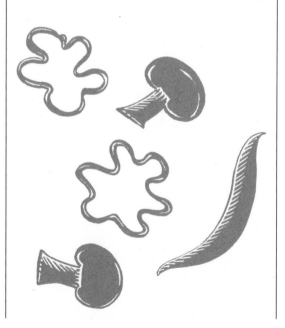

Pommes Duchesse with Almonds

A DELICIOUS WAY OF SERVING mashed potato or of re-presenting leftover potato.

INGREDIENTS

450 g (1 lb) boiled potatoes, mashed
15 g (½ oz) butter or margarine, melted
1 egg, size 1, beaten, or 2 egg yolks, beaten
15 ml (1 tbsp) ground almonds
salt and freshly ground black pepper
5 ml (1 tsp) oil
15 g (½ oz) blanched slivered almonds

SERVES 4 – 6

■ Make sure the potatoes are well mashed with no lumps, then beat in the butter well. Mix in the egg, reserving enough to brush over the top for a glaze. Mix the ground almonds thoroughly in and season to taste, mixing well.

■ Oil an ovenproof dish and put in the potato and almond mixture, then level the top. Brush with the remaining egg and scatter the slivered almonds over. Cook at 200°C (400°F) mark 6 for 20–25 minutes or until the top is golden.

4 SERVINGS		6 SERVINGS	
kcals	180	kcals	120
kJ	755	kJ	505
CHO	20 g	CHO	15 g
Fibre	2 g	Fibre	1 g

VARIATION

TO THE POTATO AND ALMOND MIXTURE, add 150 g (5 oz) cooked, drained, puréed spinach and mix in well, with an addition of a good pinch of freshly grated nutmeg to the seasoning. After glazing the top with the remaining egg and scattering over the slivered almonds, shake over 40 g (1½ oz) finely grated Parmesan cheese, dot with a few nuts of butter and bake.

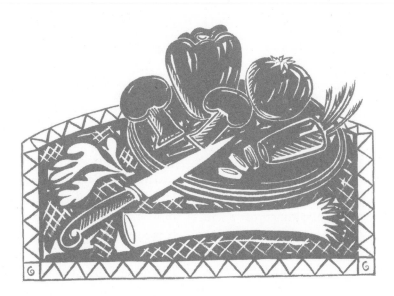

SAUCES, DRESSINGS AND STUFFINGS

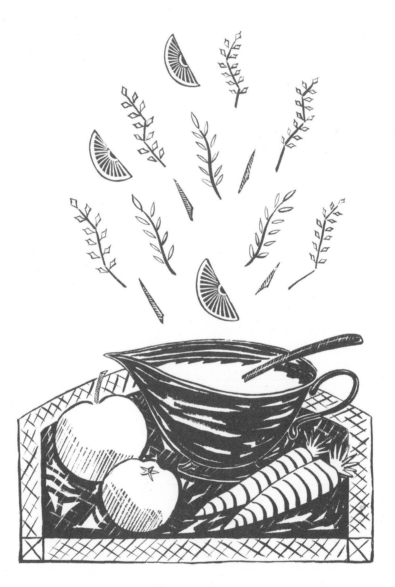

THIS CHAPTER IS AN IMPORTANT ONE in the book for although in some cases the additions mean a few more grams of CHO, it is sensible to make allowance for them. All diets, if too plain, become monotonous and it is this monotony which can cause people to wander away from them. A sauce, a dressing and a good stuffing, which add flavour, can give that fillip which makes all the difference between monotony and a welcome change of taste. It is not necessary to have large helpings of them, but just enough to bring out flavour and give a variety of taste.

Apple Sauce

SERVED WITH DUCK, pork or goose, this sauce should not be too sweet as its use is to contrast with the richness of the meats.

INGREDIENTS

450 g (1 lb) cooking apples, peeled, cored and diced
30–40 ml (3–4 tbsp) water
25 g (1 oz) butter or margarine
10 ml (2 tsp) fructose or 30–40 ml (2–3 tbsp) chopped sultanas (optional)
squeeze of fresh lemon juice, to taste

SERVES 4 – 6

▮ Put the apples into a saucepan with the water. Cook slowly, uncovered, for about 10 minutes until they are soft and form a purée when stirred. Beat into a purée, sieve or liquidise.

▮ Add the butter, fructose or sultanas and a small squeeze of lemon juice.

4 SERVINGS		6 SERVINGS	
kcals	115	kcals	75
kJ	480	kJ	320
CHO	15 g	CHO	10 g
Fibre	3 g	Fibre	2 g

VARIATION

ADD 5 ml (1 tsp) finely grated zest of lemon to the sauce at the last minute, to give an additional zing.

Beurre Noir

A SIMPLE FRENCH SAUCE which is excellent served over poached or cocotte eggs, brains or sweetbreads and, particularly, poached skate.

INGREDIENTS

175 g (6 oz) butter or margarine
45 ml (3 tbsp) capers, drained
15 ml (1 tbsp) white wine vinegar

SERVES 4

▮ Melt the butter in a heavy saucepan over a medium heat until golden brown, but be sure it does not blacken or burn.

▮ Add the capers, then the vinegar. Heat through and serve.

4 SERVINGS	
kcals	325
kJ	1335
CHO	0
Fibre	0

Avocado Sauce

A MOST DELICIOUS COLD SAUCE for almost any cold food, such as hard-boiled eggs, fish, meat or poultry. It can also be used as a dip.

INGREDIENTS

2 avocados, stoned and skinned
10 ml (2 tsp) freshly squeezed lemon juice
30–40 ml (2–3 tbsp) soured cream or natural yogurt
salt

SERVES 4

■ Blend all the ingredients for the sauce in a liquidiser or food processor until smooth.

■ Taste for seasoning and add more lemon juice or salt if needed. Cover and chill until served.

4 SERVINGS	
kcals	210
kJ	875
CHO	Negligible
Fibre	2 g

Mayonnaise

ANOTHER CLASSICAL FRENCH SAUCE which is easily made in a liquidiser or food processor. It is served with cold fish, particularly salmon, poultry, eggs and some vegetables. Stored in a glass screw-topped jar in the refrigerator, this creamy home-made mayonnaise will keep for at least a fortnight.

INGREDIENTS

2 egg yolks, without any white of egg
10 ml (2 tsp) tarragon vinegar or lemon juice
300 ml (½ pint) olive oil or half olive oil and half sunflower oil
salt
15 ml (1 tbsp) boiling water

MAKES JUST OVER 300 ml (½ pint)

■ Before starting, it is essential to have the ingredients at room temperature. The mayonnaise can be made by beating in a bowl with a wire hand whisk or, in about a quarter of the time, in a liquidiser or food processor. Particularly if using the hand whisk, it is essential to add the oil very slowly, a very little at a time.

■ Put the egg yolks into a bowl or into the container of a liquidiser or food processor. Add half the vinegar and beat or blend. While whisking or as the machine is running, slowly add the oil, a little at a time. As the sauce thickens, slightly increase the rate of adding oil, but be cautious, too much added too suddenly will cause instant 'curdling' or separating; see below.

■ When the mayonnaise has reached the consistency of butter in a hot room in summertime, add the remaining vinegar, then, slowly, a little more oil, until it thickens again. Add salt to taste, then finally the boiling water, whisking or blending vigorously.

■ If you have added the oil too fast, or started with egg yolks straight from the refrigerator and the mayonnaise has curdled, remove the mayonnaise, clean the container. Put in another egg yolk and start again, adding the curdled mayonnaise, a little at a time, as you whisk and blend energetically.

TOTAL	
kcals	2215
kJ	9120
CHO	0
Fibre	0

VARIATIONS

THERE ARE A GREAT MANY different sauces that can be made from a basic mayonnaise. For Aioli, mix 2–3 skinned, crushed and pounded garlic cloves thoroughly into each 90 ml (6 tbsp) mayonnaise. It is superb with jacket-baked potatoes, cold poached cod or with cauliflower.

Guacamole, a Mexican sauce, uses 90 ml (6 tbsp) mayonnaise, 2 puréed avocados, lemon juice, salt and a dash of Tabasco. It is excellent with hard-boiled eggs, or as a salad dressing or a dip.

For Niçoise, mix 300 ml (½ pint) mayonnaise, 1 medium red pepper, cored, deseeded and puréed, 15 ml (1 tbsp) tomato purée and 5 ml (1 tsp) finely chopped fresh tarragon. It is good with hard-boiled eggs, cold cooked chicken or fish.

For Sauce Verte, combine 300 ml (½ pint) mayonnaise with 30–40 ml (2–3 tbsp) finely chopped fresh parsley, chives and tarragon mixed. This sauce goes well with eggs, fish or poultry.

For Sauce Tartare, mix 300 ml (½ pint) mayonnaise with 15 ml (1 tbsp) chopped fresh chives, 15 ml (1 tbsp) chopped fresh parsley, 15–30 ml (1–2 tbsp) finely chopped capers, 4–5 finely chopped small gherkins and 5 ml (1 tsp) mild Dijon mustard. This sauce is essential with steak tartare, and is also excellent with cold cooked meats and hot or cold fish.

Liquidiser Hollandaise Sauce

A CLASSICAL SAUCE for hot salmon, chicken, eggs and some vegetables, such as asparagus or broccoli, though cauliflower is excellent too.

If you are delayed in serving the sauce, keep it warm over warm water in a double boiler. Whisk just before serving.

INGREDIENTS
100 g (4 oz) butter, unsalted, at room temperature
2 egg yolks
10 ml (2 tsp) freshly squeezed lemon juice or 10 ml (2 tsp) dry white wine or tarragon vinegar
salt and freshly ground white pepper
MAKES ABOUT 300 ml (½ pint)

■ Heat the butter in a saucepan until foaming, but do not allow it to brown. Put the yolks into the liquidiser, add the lemon juice, a little salt and a grind of white pepper. Cover and blend for about 2 seconds on LOW.

■ Turn to HIGH, take off the cover and slowly add the hot butter until it is all absorbed.

TOTAL	
kcals	875
kJ	3605
CHO	0
Fibre	0

VARIATION

ADDING 30 ml (2 tbsp) DOUBLE CREAM or 1 stiffly whisked egg white will convert the Hollandaise into a Sauce Mousseline.

Herb Sauce

AN EXTREMELY EASY, fragrant sauce for serving with boiled chicken or poached fish. Many different herbs can be used. For serving with poultry, a defatted chicken stock should be used; if with fish, a fish stock. For poultry, tarragon, chervil and parsley are good herbs to make predominate. When serving with fish, burnet, fennel or mint give a suitable character to the sauce, mint being particularly original and good.

INGREDIENTS
600 ml (1 pint) stock
25 g (1 oz) butter or margarine
15 ml (1 tbsp) flour
squeeze of fresh lemon juice
salt and freshly ground black pepper
30 ml (2 tbsp) chopped fresh tarragon, chervil or parsley, or for fish, burnet, fennel or mint
SERVES 4

■ If making the sauce for poultry, it is essential that the chicken stock be defatted. Heat the butter in a 1 litre (1¾ pint) saucepan, stir in the flour thoroughly and cook over moderate heat for 2 minutes, stirring.

■ Gradually add the stock, continuing to stir, bring to the boil and cook until smooth and thickened. Add the lemon juice and season to taste. Finally, stir in the chopped herbs.

4 SERVINGS	
kcals	55
kJ	235
CHO	Negligible
Fibre	0

VARIATION

AS WELL AS USING the individual herbs singly, you can vary your sauce by using different combinations of herbs.

Plum Sauce

A TRADITIONAL ENGLISH WEST COUNTRY SAUCE for lamb, ham or pork. Stoned cherries can also be used. Choose ripe fruit that needs no extra sweetening.

INGREDIENTS
450 g (1 lb) ripe red or purple plums, stoned
150 ml (¼ pint) dry cider or dry white wine
15–30 ml (1–2 tbsp) cider vinegar
15 ml (1 tbsp) finely chopped fresh mint (if with lamb)
MAKES ABOUT 750 ml (1½ pints)

■ Cook the plums in the cider and cider vinegar in a pan for about 15 minutes or until soft.

■ Blend in a liquidiser, if liked. Taste, the sauce may need 5 ml (1 tsp) fructose, but should not taste too sweet. Add the mint if using, just before serving.

TOTAL	
kcals	225
kJ	970
CHO	50 g
Fibre	10 g

White Sauce

THIS SIMPLE SAUCE IS INVALUABLE as a basis for other sauces rather than for serving on its own. It can be made with skimmed milk or with half skimmed milk and half stock.

INGREDIENTS
25 g (1 oz) butter or margarine
25 g (1 oz) flour (wholemeal gives a nuttier flavour)
300 ml ($\frac{1}{2}$ pint) skimmed milk or half skimmed milk and half chicken stock
salt and freshly ground black pepper
MAKES 300 ml ($\frac{1}{2}$ pint)

▌ Melt the butter in a saucepan until it is foaming but not turning brown. Remove from the heat and mix in the flour well. Put back on a medium heat and cook for 1 minute, stirring well, but do not allow it to brown.

▌ Gradually add the milk or milk and stock, stirring continually until the sauce is smooth and thickened. If too thick, add a little more liquid but whisk well while doing so. Season to taste. With this basis, a series of individually flavoured sauces can be made:

TOTAL	
kcals	365
kJ	1525
CHO	30 g
Fibre	2 g

Caper Sauce: Add 30 ml (2 tbsp) capers and 15 ml (1 tbsp) caper vinegar. For boiled mutton or fish.

Cheese Sauce: Stir in 45–60 ml (3–4 tbsp) grated cheese. For eggs, fish, cauliflower or other vegetables.

Curry Sauce: Add and stir well in 15 ml (1 tbsp) mild curry paste or to taste. For eggs, fish or chicken.

Egg Sauce: Add 2 mashed hard-boiled eggs and 5 ml (1 tsp) anchovy essence. For fish.

Mushroom Sauce: Add 100 g (4 oz) sliced, chopped mushrooms and simmer for 5–7 minutes. Good with hard-boiled eggs, as an omelette filling or with fish.

Mustard Sauce: Add 10 ml (2 tsp) French mustard and 10 ml (2 tsp) English mustard and stir well in. Good with grilled herrings or mackerel.

Parsley Sauce: Add 30 ml (2 tbsp) finely chopped fresh parsley and stir well in. Good with ham, boiled mutton or fish.

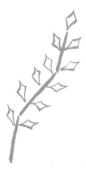

Tomato Sauce

AN EASY AND USEFUL SAUCE to enjoy poured over pasta and rice dishes or for cooking with chicken portions, chops or eggs. If made without garlic or onion, it can be frozen for months: these can be added when the sauce is required. Garlic, onion and all the allium family do not freeze well and should always be added after thawing. However, if the top of the sauce is covered with a thin layer of oil, the complete sauce can be kept for a week in the refrigerator without spoiling.

INGREDIENTS

1.8 kg (4 lb) tomatoes, skinned and chopped, or canned and drained

1 bay leaf

large pinch of dried marjoram or basil

1 small to medium red or green pepper, cored, deseeded and chopped

1 large onion, skinned and chopped (if not freezing)

2 garlic cloves, skinned and chopped (if not freezing)

150 ml ($\frac{1}{4}$ pint) juice from canned tomatoes, water or dry red wine

salt and freshly ground black pepper

MAKES ABOUT 1.4 kg (3 lb)

■ Put all the ingredients into a large saucepan, omitting the onion and garlic if intending to freeze the sauce. Bring to the boil, simmer gently for about 1 hour or until the liquid is almost absorbed and the tomatoes make a thick purée.

■ Take out the bay leaf and liquidise the sauce, or leave as it is. Tomato sauce can be bottled as for bottled fruit. Transfer the boiling sauce to sterilised glass jars. Seal at once with sterile tops.

TOTAL	
kcals	385
kJ	1640
CHO	50 g
Fibre	20 g

Vegetable Purées as Sauces

THIS IS AN IDEA which I evolved to give fat-free sauces which are delicious and easy to make. You can no doubt think of others, but here are some to start with. The vegetables are best cooked by steaming or, better still, if you have the special alloy saucepans by 'waterless' cooking. They should then be puréed in a vegetable mill or food processor. All freeze well, so it is worth storing some in containers of suitable size. Thaw out at room temperature or in the microwave oven set at DEFROST.

Celeriac purée goes very well with ham, duck, pork or salt beef. Pepper purée, using cored, deseeded, quartered and steamed peppers, are good with fish or chicken. Members of the allium family also make admirable purée sauces but do not freeze well. Leek purée is good with bacon, chicken or salt beef. Onion purée is delicious with goose or boiled mutton.

All the above should be seasoned to taste with salt and freshly ground black, green or white pepper. The addition of a little natural yogurt or soured cream gives them an enticing richness and, heated with defatted stock and skimmed milk, gives a satisfying slimmer's soup.

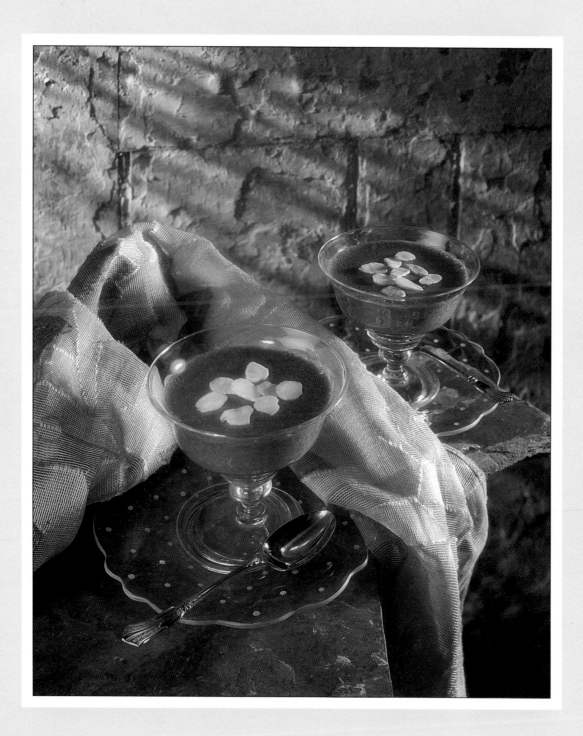

Chocolate and Coffee Mousse (page 131)

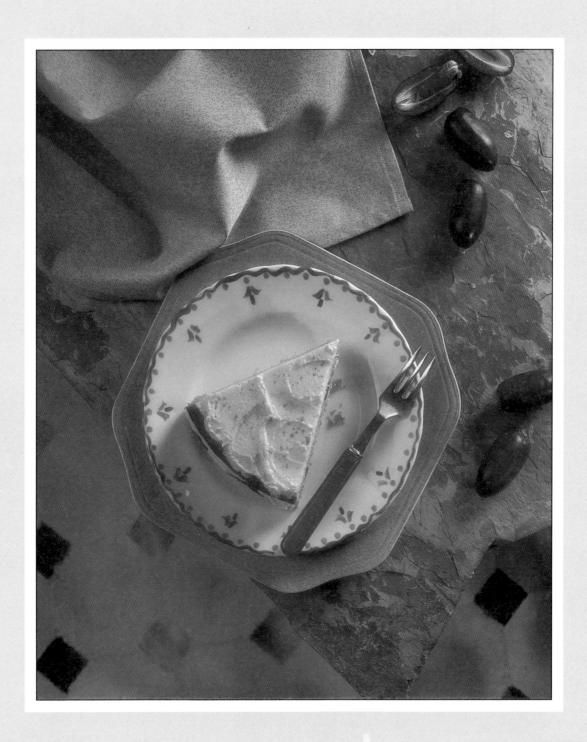

Spicy Carrot Cake (page 136)

How to Make Yogurt

MANY OF YOU MAY have appliances for yogurt making and already appreciate the great difference in both price and flavour between the home-made and commercial varieties. However, to make excellent yogurt you only need a wide-mouthed vacuum flask of 1.1 litre (2 pint) capacity, a dairy or clinical thermometer and to take a very small amount of care with milk temperatures.

INGREDIENTS
1.1 litres (2 pints) milk, skimmed or full cream
20 ml (4 tsp) fresh natural yogurt
MAKES 1.1 litres (2 pints)

■ Put the milk into a deep saucepan, bring to the boil and boil for 1 minute. It is handy to have one of those little glass discs that prevent the milk from foaming up suddenly in the saucepan. If you do not have one, just watch the milk more carefully as it comes to the boil, preventing it boiling over by reducing the heat.

■ Take from the heat after 1 minute and pour the milk into a large stainless steel or aluminium jug and immerse the lower half in cold water until the milk has cooled to just between 42–43°C (105–108°F) as shown on the thermometer. **It is essential that the milk is neither hotter nor cooler than this**. Lift the jug out of the cold water and at once whisk in the yogurt thoroughly.

■ Pour the mixture into the vacuum flask, seal and leave overnight. If the yogurt was fresh, you will have 1.1 litres (2 pints) well set yogurt.

TOTAL	
kcals	375
kJ	1605
CHO	55 g
Fibre	0

Yogurt Spiced Sauce

KNOWN AS *Sughtoror Madzoon*, this is one of the most popular sauces throughout the Middle East. It accompanies vegetable dishes, kebabs and stews.

INGREDIENTS
300 ml (½ pint) natural yogurt, preferably Greek strained yogurt
1–2 garlic cloves, skinned and crushed
1.25 ml (¼ tsp) salt
1.25 ml (¼ tsp) ground cumin
1.25 ml (¼ tsp) ground cinnamon
5 ml (1 tsp) finely chopped fresh mint
1 spring onion, trimmed and chopped (optional)
MAKES 300 ml (½ pint)

■ Pour the yogurt into a bowl, add the garlic and mix well. Add the spices, stirring well. Chill.

■ A few minutes before serving, take from the refrigerator, put into a cold serving bowl, sprinkle with the mint and spring onion if using, and serve.

TOTAL	
kcals	170
kJ	705
CHO	20 g
Fibre	0

Yogurt Dressing

A CREAMY YOGURT MADE from full cream milk is best for this. It is good with salads of all kinds as well as hard-boiled eggs.

INGREDIENTS
300 ml (½ pint) natural yogurt
10 ml (2 tsp) olive or sunflower oil
10 ml (2 tsp) freshly squeezed lemon juice or cider vinegar
1–2 garlic cloves, skinned and crushed
salt
MAKES ABOUT 300 ml (½ pint)

■ Beat all the ingredients together, adding the garlic and salt last, to taste. Do not make this dressing too long in advance as it has a tendency to separate if left standing for a long time.

TOTAL	
kcals	220
kJ	910
CHO	20 g
Fibre	0

French Dressing or Vinaigrette

THIS OIL AND VINEGAR DRESSING is perhaps the most common and the most useful of any. I prefer it made with olive oil, but everyone's taste varies. I also like the simple French version, without mustard or sweetening. The usual proportions are between 3–4 parts oil to 1 part wine vinegar, though there are some occasions, such as a tomato salad for example, when a higher proportion of vinegar can be good. There is no difficulty about varying the proportions to suit your inclination, but too much vinegar makes the oil separate rapidly. A vinaigrette should never be put on to a salad until just before it is going to be eaten. If the salad is covered in water droplets, this will de-stabilise the dressing, so green salads in particular should always be dried first.

INGREDIENTS
60 ml (4 tbsp) olive or sunflower oil
15 ml (1 tbsp) white or red wine vinegar or tarragon vinegar
salt and freshly ground black pepper
SERVES 4

■ Put the oil, vinegar and seasoning into a bowl or tight screw-topped glass jar. Whisk briskly or shake vigorously until an emulsion is formed.

4 SERVINGS	
kcals	110
kJ	445
CHO	0
Fibre	0

VARIATIONS

IN FRANCE, where a fine wine is to be served, the vinegar in the dressing is replaced by a dry white or red wine or, sometimes, by lemon juice.

If you like the flavour of mustard in a vinaigrette, add 2.5 ml (½ tsp) Dijon mustard before shaking or whisking.

The addition of 25 g (1 oz) crumbled Roquefort or other blue cheese, well beaten or shaken into the mixture, is popular in America.

Tahiniyeh

AN IMPORTANT ARAB DRESSING and sauce from Syria and the Lebanon. It is used with some salads and as a delicious dip. Its principle ingredient is tahina, a cream made from ground sesame seeds, which can now be bought from most good Middle East grocers in our larger cities or from good health food shops.

INGREDIENTS

150 ml ($\frac{1}{4}$ pint) tahina paste
freshly squeezed juice of 2 lemons
300 ml ($\frac{1}{2}$ pint) milk or water
2 garlic cloves, skinned and crushed
15 ml (1 tbsp) finely chopped fresh parsley
5 ml (1 tsp) salt
pinch of ground chilli
MAKES 200 ml ($\frac{1}{3}$ pint)

▪ Put the tahina in a bowl and stir in the lemon juice well. Slowly add the milk, stirring continually to ensure that the mixture is even and creamy.

▪ Add the remaining ingredients and mix well. Covered, it will keep for several days in the refrigerator.

TOTAL	
kcals	1100
kJ	4615
CHO	30 g
Fibre	10 g

Soured Cream Dressing

A SIMPLE YET DELICIOUS DRESSING to serve with smoked fish, such as buckling, mackerel or trout or with marinated herring. It is also good with mushrooms, either raw and peeled or lightly poached, and excellent with potato salad and on hot jacket potatoes.

INGREDIENTS

175 ml (6 fl oz) soured cream
5–10 ml (1–2 tsp) freshly squeezed lemon juice
salt
SERVES ABOUT 3

▪ Mix the soured cream thoroughly with the lemon juice and add salt to taste.

3 SERVINGS	
kcals	105
kJ	435
CHO	Negligible
Fibre	0

VARIATIONS

WITH 5–10 ml (1–2 tsp) STRONG GROUND horseradish made up with a little water and well mixed in, it makes the best horseradish sauce ever.

With 15 ml (1 tbsp) finely chopped fresh chives, chervil or mint and a skinned and crushed garlic clove, it is surpassingly good over jacket baked potatoes.

Carrot and Apple Purée

THIS IS EXCELLENT with cooked ham, bacon or salt beef.

INGREDIENTS

450 g (1 lb) carrots, scraped, steamed, drained and puréed

2 large eating apples, peeled, cored, steamed and puréed

SERVES ABOUT 4

▪ Mix the carrots and apples together.

4 SERVINGS	
kcals	70
kJ	305
CHO	20 g
Fibre	5 g

Traditional Sausagemeat Stuffing

A GOOD STUFFING FOR MEATS or vegetables, and especially for the turkey body.

INGREDIENTS

100 g (4 oz) rashers streaky bacon, derinded and chopped

15 g (½ oz) butter or soft margarine

1 large onion, skinned and finely chopped

900 g (2 lb) fresh pork sausagemeat

5 ml (1 tsp) finely chopped fresh rosemary or ground sage

salt and freshly ground black pepper

ENOUGH FOR A 5.5–6.8 kg (12–15 lb) TURKEY

▪ Put the bacon with the butter in a pan and, when the butter has melted, add the onion and soften but do not allow it to colour.

▪ Mix the sausagemeat and rosemary in a bowl and add the onion and bacon, mixing well. Season to taste.

TOTAL	
kcals	3860
kJ	15980
CHO	90 g
Fibre	3 g

VARIATION

FOR A CHANGE, shape this mixture into small balls and fry or bake separately.

Chestnut Stuffing

A FINE TRADITIONAL STUFFING for turkey or game.

INGREDIENTS

700 g (1½ lb) Spanish chestnuts, shelled and skinned, or 450 g (1 lb) canned, unsweetened, whole chestnuts, drained

50 g (2 oz) fresh sausagemeat

salt and freshly ground black pepper

25 g (1 oz) butter or margarine

ENOUGH FOR THE CROP OF A 5.4–6.3 kg (12–14 lb) TURKEY

▪ If using fresh chestnuts, make a slit in one side of each nut. Boil them in a pan of water for 30 minutes or until a thin pronged fork will just penetrate. While they are hot, shell them and remove the inner skin, one at a time, discarding any that are not sound.

■ Mix the nuts with the other ingredients. The nuts need not be mashed and should be mostly whole. Add enough butter to bind the stuffing.

■ If using canned whole chestnuts the procedure is the same but mix gently to keep as many whole as possible. Any left over can be rolled into small balls, and fried or baked and served around the bird.

TOTAL	
kcals	1550
kJ	6530
CHO	260 g
Fibre	48 g

VARIATION

ABOUT 25 g (1 oz) wholemeal breadcrumbs and an egg yolk can be used instead of sausagemeat. A chestnut purée for serving with game can be made with mashed cooked chestnuts mixed with 15–30 ml (1–2 tbsp) consommé and seasoning.

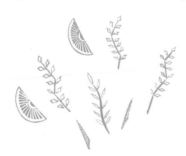

Skirlie or Oatmeal Stuffing

A MOST DELICIOUS AND EASY Scottish stuffing for all poultry, boiled or roasted meats or ham. It can also be made into a savoury pudding to be served with meat or fish.

INGREDIENTS
100 g (4 oz) medium oatmeal, lightly toasted
1 medium to large onion, skinned and finely chopped
45 ml (3 tbsp) melted butter, margarine or, traditionally, grated suet
pinch of chopped parsley
pinch of chopped thyme
30 ml (2 tbsp) stock, preferably giblet, or, for special occasions, whisky
salt and freshly ground white pepper

ENOUGH FOR A 1.8 kg (4 lb) BIRD

■ To toast the oatmeal lightly, shake out on to a baking sheet and brown in a moderate oven or under a moderate grill. Turn the oatmeal and make sure it does not blacken.

■ Transfer to a bowl and add the other ingredients in the order given, mixing well. Stuff both the crop and the body of the bird and secure well with small skewers.

TOTAL	
kcals	770
kJ	3225
CHO	80 g
Fibre	10 g

VARIATIONS

SKIRLIE CAN BE ROLLED into small balls and poached like dumplings in boiling soup, particularly Scotch broth, see page 27.

For a savoury pudding, put all the mixed ingredients into a greased pudding basin, cover to exclude the water and steam or boil for 1 hour. Serve with meats, game or cod with mustard sauce.

Apricot and Almond Stuffing

AN UNUSUAL BUT DELICIOUS STUFFING for any poultry or pork.

INGREDIENTS

50 g (2 oz) soft margarine or butter
1 large onion, skinned and chopped
225 g (8 oz) dried apricots, soaked for at least 4 hours, drained and chopped
100 g (4 oz) ground almonds
30 ml (2 tbsp) sultanas
5 ml (1 tsp) finely grated orange rind
pinch of ground cinnamon
30 ml (2 tbsp) fresh orange juice, strained
salt and freshly ground black pepper

ENOUGH FOR A 1.4–1.6 kg (3–3½ lb) BIRD

◼ Heat the margarine in a pan and soften the onion but do not allow it to colour. Add the apricots and heat for 2 minutes, mixing well.

◼ Drain off excess fat, transfer to a bowl and mix in all the remaining ingredients. If it seems too dry and crumbly, add a little more orange juice.

TOTAL	
kcals	1445
kJ	6030
CHO	125 g
Fibre	72 g

Celery and Walnut Stuffing

ANOTHER EXCELLENT STUFFING which gives good flavour to poultry and meats, especially lamb.

INGREDIENTS

50 g (2 oz) wholemeal breadcrumbs
75 g (3 oz) ground walnuts
1 celery heart, trimmed and finely chopped
pinch of ground cinnamon
pinch of ground ginger
5 ml (1 tsp) dried tarragon
5 ml (1 tsp) grated lemon rind
5 ml (1 tsp) lemon juice
salt and freshly ground black pepper
15–30 ml (1–2 tbsp) unsweetened apple juice or stock

ENOUGH FOR A 1.4–1.6 kg (3–3½ lb) BIRD

◼ Mix all the stuffing ingredients together. Moisten with enough apple juice to give a malleable texture.

TOTAL	
kcals	535
kJ	2225
CHO	30 g
Fibre	10 g

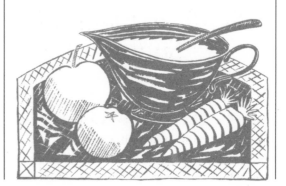

BAKING

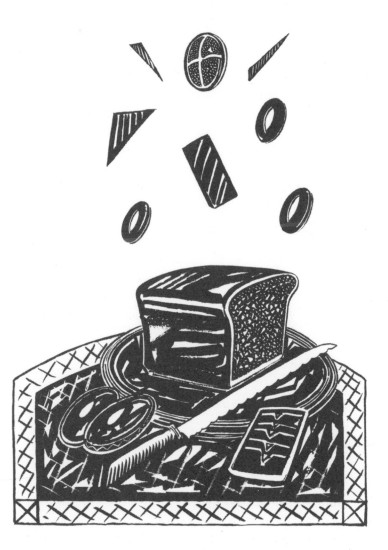

GOOD BROWN BREAD is sometimes difficult to find and usually expensive. It is not difficult to make your own, with or without yeast, and it freezes very well. Therefore it is an excellent idea to bake several loaves at the same time and freeze those you won't be using immediately.

Sugar-free teabreads are harder to find in shops than good bread and when found are often very dry and not worth the money. Those on the following pages are made regularly in my household and devoured by everyone. Sugar is not an essential food for anyone and even those of us who are non-diabetic will often profit by avoiding it. The same applies to scones and biscuits, both of which store very well.

Wholemeal pastry is just as easy to make as that made with white flour. If you find that the family doesn't like it as much, then begin gradually by adding part wholemeal to the white, until they have got accustomed to wholemeal pastry. It is best to start using the wholemeal with savoury dishes as it gives a fine, slightly nutty taste.

Wholemeal Yeast Bread

INGREDIENTS

5 ml (1 tsp) fructose
250 ml (9 fl oz) lukewarm water
7.5 ml (1½ tsp) dried or 15 g (½ oz) fresh yeast*
450 g (1 lb) wholemeal flour
5 ml (1 tsp) salt
15 ml (1 tbsp) polyunsaturated margarine or sunflower oil
25 mg vitamin C, if using fresh yeast by the quick method*

MAKES A 450 g (1 lb) LOAF

*The use of vitamin C (laevo-ascorbic acid) with fresh yeast, can reduce the proving time by more than half. Conveniently available in 25 mg tablets, one tablet should be crushed and dissolved in the lukewarm water at the same time as the fructose. This method does not work with dried yeasts.

■ Dissolve the fructose (and the crushed vitamin C tablet if using fresh yeast) in the lukewarm water. Stir in the yeast and leave for 10–15 minutes in a warm place until frothing commences.

■ If you have a kneading machine or a food processor, follow the instruction booklet. Alternatively, mix the flour and salt in a large bowl and rub in the margarine or mix in the oil. Mix the yeast liquid well into the flour to form a dough.

■ Turn out on to a lightly floured surface and knead by slightly flattening the dough, folding it towards you and pressing it down. Fold the sides into the centre, press down again, then turn the dough through 90 degrees. Repeat the operation over and over until the dough has become uniform, firm and elastic in texture.

■ Put the dough into a large bowl and the bowl into a polythene bag large enough to leave room for expansion. Put in a warm place for the first proving, closing the bag to keep the carbon dioxide, produced by the yeast, from dissipating. Leave until the dough has doubled in size; for dried yeast will be about 1½ hours and for fresh yeast with vitamin C less than half this time.

■ When the dough has doubled in volume, turn it out on to a lightly floured surface and knead, as before, for about 2 minutes. Shape the dough to fit a lightly greased or oiled 450 g (1 lb) loaf tin and put into the tin. Put the tin into the bag, close the bag and leave in a warm place for about a further 45 minutes until the dough has just begun to become round above the rim of the tin. This will take less time with fresh yeast and vitamin C.

■ When the dough is ready, remove the bag and make a score along the centre to ensure even tension in the crust. Bake at 230°C (450°F) mark 8 for the first 15 minutes, then lower the oven temperature to 200°C (400°F) mark 6 and bake for a further 20–30 minutes until the top is a golden brown. Run a knife around inside the edges of the tin and turn out the loaf on to a wire rack to cool. If completely cooked, the bottom will sound hollow when tapped. (As flours and ovens vary greatly, even today, these baking times can only be a fairly accurate guide which you can refine from your own practical experience.)

PER 25 g (1 oz) SLICE	
kcals	55
kJ	230
CHO	10 g
Fibre	2 g

VARIATIONS

WHITE BREAD or bread made from half wholemeal and half white flour can be made in the same way, but the white variety will tend to need a slightly shorter baking time. Remember too, that the white loaf will, because it has less fibre content, have a higher CHO value in a weight for weight comparison with the wholemeal. Add 75 g (3 oz) dried fruit during mixing if liked.

To make rolls: after the final kneading, divide the dough into 12 and shape into small rolls. Place, well separated, on a lightly floured baking sheet, place in a large polythene bag. Inflate the bag so that it does not come in contact with the dough and knot it to keep it inflated while the final proving takes place. When ready, remove the bag and bake as before for about 25 minutes.

Irish Farmhouse Loaf

A DELICIOUS FRUIT LOAF containing oatmeal as well as flour.

INGREDIENTS
350 g (12 oz) wholemeal self-raising flour
100 g (4 oz) oatmeal
5 ml (1 tsp) baking powder
pinch of bicarbonate of soda
5 ml (1 tsp) salt
10–15 ml (2–3 tsp) ground mixed spice
15 ml (1 tbsp) fructose
grated rind of $\frac{1}{2}$ lemon
75 g (3 oz) mixed dried fruit
1 egg, size 2, beaten
300 ml ($\frac{1}{2}$ pint) buttermilk or 300 ml ($\frac{1}{2}$ pint) natural yogurt
150 ml ($\frac{1}{4}$ pint) water

MAKES ABOUT A 900 g (2 lb) LOAF, 20 AVERAGE SLICES

■ Mix all the dry ingredients together in a bowl and add the lemon rind and dried fruit. Beat the egg into the buttermilk or yogurt and water. Mix well into the other ingredients to make a good, soft and elastic dough.

■ Turn out the dough on to a lightly floured surface and knead a little. Shape to fit a lightly greased 900 g (2 lb) loaf tin. Put into the loaf tin, making sure the corners are well filled. Bake at 200°C (400°F) mark 6 for 45 minutes to 1 hour. Cool on a wire rack.

PER SLICE	
kcals	90
kJ	390
CHO	20 g
Fibre	2 g

Never-Fail Soda Bread

THIS MAKES AN EXCELLENT LOAF and, when baked in a loaf tin, cuts into slices more easily. If made with all wholemeal flour, the texture is coarser.

INGREDIENTS
225 g (8 oz) wholemeal flour
225 g (8 oz) plain white flour
15 ml (1 tbsp) wheat germ
6.25 ml (1¼ tsp) bicarbonate of soda or 5 ml (1 tsp) bicarbonate of soda if using buttermilk
15 ml (1 tbsp) baking powder
10 ml (2 tsp) salt
pinch of ground coriander or ginger
1 egg, size 2, beaten
450 ml (¾ pint) buttermilk or 300 ml (½ pint) natural yogurt and 150 ml (¼ pint) water
MAKES A 900 g (2 lb) LOAF

■ Sift all the dry ingredients together into a large bowl. Beat the egg into the buttermilk or yogurt and water mixture. Make a 'well' in the centre of the dry ingredients and pour the liquid in, mixing thoroughly to form a consistent dough.

■ Turn out the dough on to a lightly floured surface and knead for a few minutes until pliable. Either shape by hand into round, flattish loaves or put into a lightly greased 900 g (2 lb) loaf tin. Score a cross on the top to ensure an even tension in the crust. Bake at 190°C (375°F) mark 5 for about 35 minutes. Cool on a wire rack. Wrap the soda bread in a tea-towel to keep the crust from getting hard and stale.

PER 25 g (1 oz) SLICE	
kcals	70
kJ	295
CHO	15 g
Fibre	1 g

VARIATIONS

SMALL ROLLS CAN BE MADE from the dough. Put on to a lightly greased and floured baking sheet and bake for about 20 minutes. Cool on a wire rack and store in an airtight tin as they go stale quickly.

About 50 g (2 oz) raisins or sultanas can be added to the dough if liked.

Wholemeal Apple Scones

THESE ARE DELICIOUS spread with cottage cheese or quark, or with a hard cheese. The flavour is tart.

INGREDIENTS
225 g (8 oz) wholemeal flour
20 ml (4 tsp) baking powder
pinch of salt
50 g (2 oz) butter or polyunsaturated margarine
30 ml (2 tbsp) peeled, grated cooking apple
150 ml (¼ pint) skimmed milk
1 egg, size 2, beaten
MAKES ABOUT 8 – 10

■ Mix the dry ingredients well together in a bowl. Rub in the butter and stir in the apple. Beat the milk and egg together and add to the mixture gradually to form a manageable dough. Reserve any milk and egg mixture left over for glazing.

▌ Turn out the dough on to a lightly floured surface and knead very lightly. Roll out the dough into a sheet 1 cm ($\frac{1}{2}$ inch) thick and cut into 5 cm (2 inch) rounds. Alternatively, form the dough into one large flat round and mark from the centre into 8 triangles. Put on a lightly greased baking sheet and brush over the top with the remaining milk and egg mixture.

▌ Bake at 200°C (400°F) mark 6 for 10–12 minutes for single scones or the large round for 15–20 minutes.

8 SCONES		10 SCONES	
kcals	160	kcals	130
kJ	675	kJ	540
CHO	20 g	CHO	15 g
Fibre	3 g	Fibre	2 g

VARIATIONS

SPICED SCONES CAN BE MADE by omitting the apple and adding 7.5 ml (1$\frac{1}{2}$ tsp) mixed spice to the dry ingredients.

Add 30–45 ml (2–3 tbsp) bran or wheat germ to the dry ingredients to make bran or wheat germ scones.

Adding 30 ml (2 tbsp) dried, soaked, chopped apricots in place of the apple gives most delicious apricot flavoured scones.

Orange Sultana Scones

THESE DELIGHTFUL SCONES are best eaten on the day they are made.

INGREDIENTS

225 g (8 oz) wholemeal self-raising flour
1.25 ml ($\frac{1}{4}$ tsp) bicarbonate of soda
50 g (2 oz) butter or margarine
100 g (4 oz) sultanas
65 ml (2$\frac{1}{2}$ fl oz) freshly squeezed orange juice
65 ml (2$\frac{1}{2}$ fl oz) skimmed milk
5 ml (1 tsp) grated orange rind
little beaten egg or milk, to glaze

MAKES ABOUT 8

▌ Mix the dry ingredients together in a bowl. Rub in the butter until the mixture is like coarse breadcrumbs. Add the remaining ingredients in the order given, mixing with the fingertips, to give a workable dough.

▌ Turn out the dough on to a floured surface and knead lightly. Roll out to a thickness of 2.5 cm (1 inch) and cut into rounds. Put the scones on to a lightly floured baking sheet and brush the tops with a little beaten egg or milk. Bake at 200°C (400°F) mark 6 for 15–20 minutes until risen and golden.

PER SCONE	
kcals	175
kJ	730
CHO	30 g
Fibre	4 g

Potato Scones

ALSO KNOWN AS POTATO CAKES, these traditional Irish favourites are often eaten hot from the oven, with butter, when their flavour is at its finest. This dough can also be used to line or cover a dish for a savoury flan.

INGREDIENTS
225 g (8 oz) self-raising flour, either half wholemeal and half white or all white
50 g (2 oz) butter or margarine, at room temperature
pinch of salt
175 g (6 oz) cooked potato, freshly mashed or freshly made 'instant' potato
45–60 ml (3–4 tbsp) milk
MAKES 9

▮ Mix the flour with the butter in a bowl and add a good pinch of salt. Combine with the mashed potato, adding enough milk to make a soft, slack dough.

▮ Turn out the dough on to a lightly floured surface and roll out to about 2.5 cm (1 inch) thickness. Cut into rounds 5–6.5 cm (2–2½ inches) in diameter. Put the scones on to a lightly greased baking sheet. Bake at 220°C (425°F) mark 7 for 20–30 minutes. Serve hot, split in half, with butter.

PER SCONE	
kcals	140
kJ	595
CHO	20 g
Fibre	2 g

VARIATION

ROLL OUT THE DOUGH to a thickness of 1 cm (½ inch) and make rounds of about 18 cm (7 inch) diameter or cut into triangles of the same area. Prick these all over on both sides and fry them in bacon fat for 2–3 minutes on each side. Called *Fadge* in the North of Ireland, they are usually served at breakfast with bacon and eggs.

Carob and Raisin Teabread

WHEN COOKED, carob powder or flour has a chocolate-like flavour with a hint of cinnamon. It is made from the carob or locust bean. Growing on trees, these are the beans which, with wild honey, are said to have sustained St. John the Baptist in the wilderness, and very nutritious they are. The flour made from them is still known in parts of Europe as 'St. John's Bread'.

INGREDIENTS
175 g (6 oz) raisins
150 ml (¼ pint) skimmed milk
50 g (2 oz) butter, softened, or polyunsaturated margarine
2 eggs, size 1, beaten
60 ml (4 tbsp) sunflower oil
150 g (5 oz) wholemeal self-raising flour
25 g (1 oz) carob flour or powder
50 g (2 oz) fine oatmeal
MAKES A 900 g (2 lb) LOAF, ABOUT 12 SLICES

■ Put the raisins, milk, butter, eggs and oil into a bowl and blend together well until smooth and creamy. Mix the wholemeal flour, carob flour and oatmeal together in a separate bowl, then stir in the raisin mixture.

■ Spoon the mixture into an oiled and lined 900 g (2 lb) loaf tin or use a non-stick one. Level the top. Bake at 180°C (350°F) mark 4 for about 1 hour. Cool on a wire rack, then remove the lining paper.

PER SLICE	
kcals	195
kJ	815
CHO	25 g
Fibre	3 g

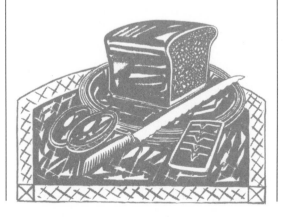

Rhubarb and Date Teabread

AN UNUSUAL COMBINATION which has a cake-like quality.

INGREDIENTS
225 g (8 oz) rhubarb, trimmed and chopped
225 g (8 oz) wholemeal flour
15 ml (1 tbsp) baking powder
50 g (2 oz) butter or margarine
175 g (6 oz) dates, stoned and finely chopped
1 egg, size 1, beaten
60 ml (4 tbsp) skimmed milk

MAKES ABOUT 12 SLICES

■ Cook the rhubarb in only 30 ml (2 tbsp) water until a purée and all the water is absorbed.

■ Put the flour and baking powder into a bowl and mix well. Rub in the butter, then stir in the rhubarb and dates. Beat the egg with the milk and combine with the rhubarb and date mixture, mixing well. Put the mixture into a 15 cm (6 inch) non-stick cake tin or a greased and lined 450 g (1 lb) loaf tin. Level the top.

■ Bake at 190°C (375°F) mark 5 for about 1 hour. Cool on a wire rack, removing any lining paper.

PER SLICE	
kcals	135
kJ	575
CHO	20 g
Fibre	4 g

VARIATION

GOOSEBERRIES, trimmed, can be used in place of the rhubarb.

Crunchy Peanut Butter Biscuits

TOAST SESAME SEEDS in a dry frying pan until golden.

INGREDIENTS
150 g (5 oz) wholemeal self-raising flour
25 g (1 oz) butter or margarine
45 ml (3 tbsp) corn oil
50 g (2 oz) crunchy peanut butter
30 ml (2 tbsp) unsweetened apple or pineapple juice
30 ml (2 tbsp) sesame seeds, toasted
MAKES ABOUT 12

■ Put the flour into a bowl and rub in the butter and oil. Add the peanut butter and apple juice, mix well. Press together with the fingers to form a pliable dough.

■ Roll out thinly on a lightly floured surface and cut into rounds or oblongs, using a 6.5 cm (2½ inch) cutter. Sprinkle with the sesame seeds. Put on to a greased baking sheet.

■ Bake at 180°C (350°F) mark 4 for 12–15 minutes. Allow to cool on the baking sheet for 5 minutes to firm, then transfer to a wire rack to cool completely.

PER BISCUIT	
kcals	120
kJ	500
CHO	10 g
Fibre	2 g

Wholemeal Pastry

WHOLEMEAL PASTRY is made as for pastry with white flour but, sometimes, slightly more cold water is needed for mixing.

For wholemeal shortcrust pastry, use twice the weight of wholemeal plain flour as fat, either butter or vegetable margarine, and just enough water to make a pliable but not slack dough. Always leave in a cool place for 30 minutes before rolling out. Cook at 200°C (400°F) mark 6 for about 25–30 minutes.

Wholemeal Flaky Pastry

THIS IS NO MORE DIFFICULT to make than when using white flour. Wholemeal flaky pastry has much more flavour and is better, dietetically, for diabetics.

INGREDIENTS
175 g (6 oz) wholemeal plain flour
pinch of salt
175 g (6 oz) softened butter or polyunsaturated margarine
squeeze of fresh lemon juice
ice-cold water, to mix
SUFFICIENT TO COVER A 20 cm (8 inch) DISH

■ Put the flour and salt into a bowl and rub in 25 g (1 oz) of the butter. Add the lemon juice and just enough cold water to make an elastic, manageable dough that can be rolled into a ball. Dust with a sprinkling of flour and turn on to a lightly floured surface.

■ Divide the remaining butter in half. Roll out the dough into a rectangle and, using half the butter, put small pieces of butter evenly over two-thirds of the area of dough nearest to you. Fold over the unbuttered third towards you, then fold the remaining buttered third over. Turn the dough through 90 degrees, then roll out into a similar rectangle. Fold into thirds again. Repeat this rolling and folding operation twice more, without butter, each time turning the dough through 90 degrees before rolling out. Wrap the dough in greaseproof paper and chill for 20–30 minutes.

▮ Roll out the chilled dough into a rectangle again and proceed in the same way with the remainder of the butter. Wrap and chill again for another 30 minutes.

▮ The dough is now ready for use. However, it will keep, wrapped, for 3 days in the refrigerator. When using, brush the surface of the dough with a little beaten egg to glaze. Bake at 220°C (425°F) mark 7 for 40–45 minutes.

TOTAL	
kcals	1850
kJ	7750
CHO	115 g
Fibre	17 g

45 ml (3 tbsp) soya oil	
35–40 ml (7–8 tsp) cold water	
TO FIT A 20 cm (8 inch) FLAN DISH	

▮ Mix the wholemeal and soya flour together in a bowl. Rub in the butter and oil until the mixture resembles breadcrumbs. Add the water and press together to form a consistent dough. Chill for 30 minutes.

▮ Roll out on a lightly floured surface and fit to the oiled flan dish. (See page 136 for a fruit flan using this pastry.)

TOTAL	
kcals	1660
kJ	6935
CHO	125 g
Fibre	23 g

Wholemeal Shortcrust Pastry with Soya Oil

THIS MAKES AN EXCELLENT PASTRY for fruit tarts or quiches. It can be eaten hot or cold.

INGREDIENTS
175 g (6 oz) wholemeal plain flour
50 g (2 oz) soya flour
75 g (3 oz) butter or margarine, cut into small pieces

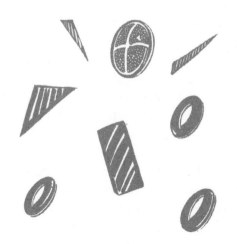

PUDDINGS

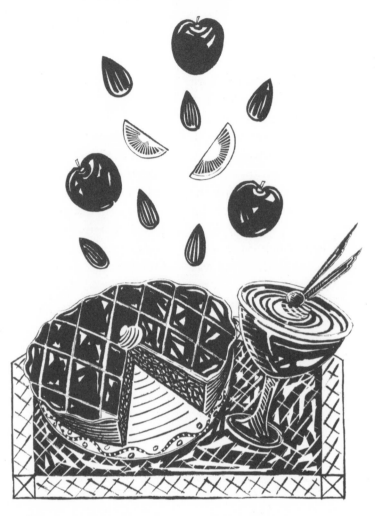

WHEN THE SUMMER FRUITS ARE AVAILABLE, there is no shortage of ideas for puddings. Orange juice, a natural sweetener, complements most soft fruits, making them even more delicious, softening the sharp edge of some, though others will be sweet enough with very little. It provides a natural ingredient either for serving fresh in a fruit salad, or for baking the firmer, larger fruits such as apples, bananas, nectarines, peaches or pears.

Fructose is very sweet and should be used cautiously, as not more than 25 g (1 oz) should be taken in 24 hours. If you have a weight problem, it is best to stick just to the fresh fruit, or some of the good sugar-free yogurts now available.

There is also a really excellent, sorbet-like pudding, in several varieties, called *Vitari*, which has a really fine flavour, contains 99% fruit and 1% natural vegetable stabiliser and absolutely nothing else—no dyes, no added sweetener of any kind and no fat. It is diabetically approved; a 75 g (3 oz) serving equals 2 fruit exchanges, i.e. 20 g CHO. It contains 97 calories per 100 g (4 oz).

If some of the recipes are not sweet enough for other members of the family, put the sugar bowl on the table so they can help themselves.

I have included a few cakes in this chapter, as they can make acceptable puddings—but watch out for the calories!

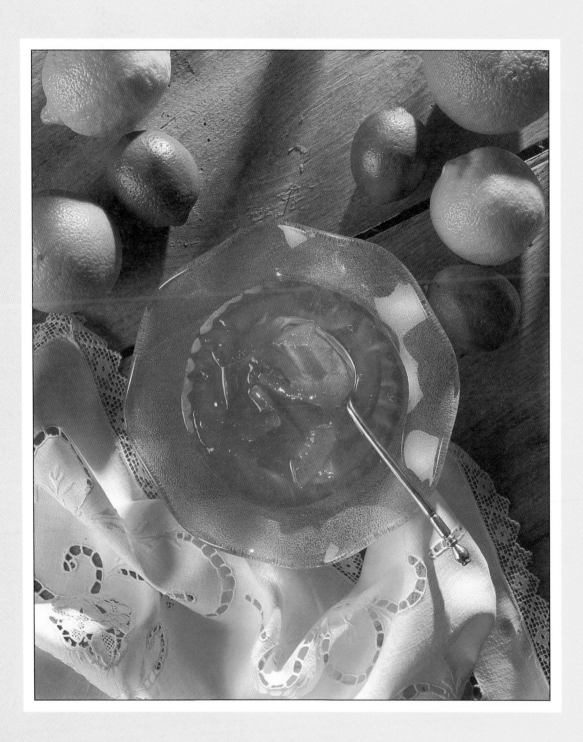

Thick Cut Dundee Marmalade (page 142)

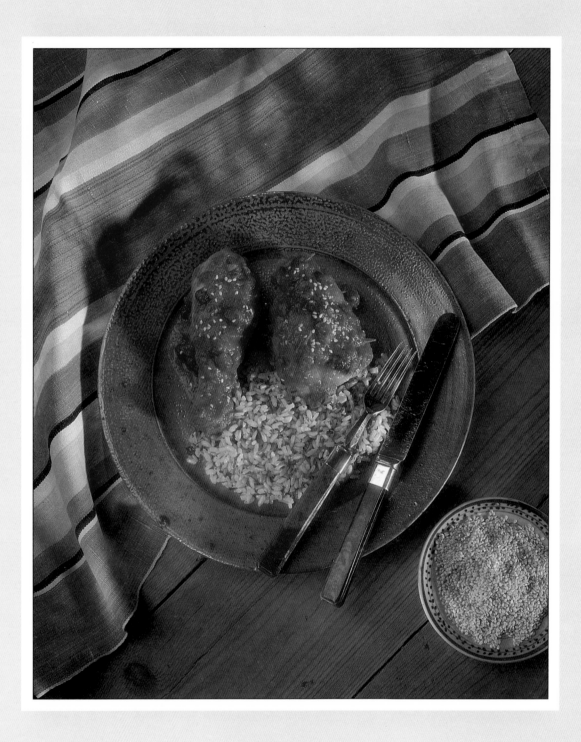

Djej Matisha Mesla (page 62)

Caledonia Ice

THIS IS A SCOTTISH RECIPE, traditionally served at harvest time or on other festive occasions at warmer times of the year. In spite of its name, it was not frozen but simply set in a cool place. The original recipe uses all double cream, which makes it very rich; I prefer a variation using curd cheese or quark.

INGREDIENTS
175 ml (6 fl oz) double cream
225 g (8 oz) curd cheese or quark
1.25 ml (¼ tsp) vanilla essence
15 ml (1 tbsp) fructose (optional)
60 ml (4 tbsp) coarse oatmeal
SERVES 4 – 6

▊ Whip the cream until stiff but not buttery. Mash the cheese and combine with the cream. Stir in the vanilla essence. Sweeten with the fructose, if using. Put into a freezerproof container, leaving a 2.5 cm (1 inch) headspace, and freeze for about 1 hour until the edges are crystallised.

▊ Meanwhile, lightly toast the oatmeal on a baking sheet in a slow oven for about 45 minutes, or under a low grill, until dried, slightly crisp but not browned.

▊ Transfer the semi-frozen cream mixture into a large bowl and mix in the toasted oatmeal thoroughly. Freeze again until solid.

▊ Remove the ice from the freezer to the refrigerator 30 minutes before serving.

4 SERVINGS		6 SERVINGS	
kcals	335	kcals	220
kJ	1390	kJ	920
CHO	10 g	CHO	5 g
Fibre	1 g	Fibre	1 g

VARIATIONS

ADD 100 g (4 oz) raspberries, puréed and sieved, or other soft fruit, at the same time as the oatmeal.

Or layer the cheese and cream mixture with whole fresh raspberries or halved strawberries, topping with the cream mixture decorated with a few of the whole fruits.

Other flavouring essences such as rum or orange can be used in place of vanilla at your discretion.

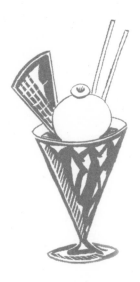

Apricot and Orange Coupe

DRIED, CANNED OR FRESH APRICOTS can be used to make this dessert.

INGREDIENTS

225 g (8 oz) dried apricots, soaked overnight, or 400 g (14 oz) canned, stoned and drained, or fresh apricots, cooked and stoned

grated rind of 1 orange

100 ml (6½ tbsp) freshly squeezed orange juice

50 g (2 oz) low-fat curd cheese or quark

30 ml (2 tbsp) low-fat natural yogurt

15 g (½ oz) flaked almonds

SERVES 4 – 6

■ Cook the apricots in the water in which they were soaked, making it up to 300 ml (½ pint) with water if needed, for about 20 minutes or until soft. Add the grated orange rind and three-quarters of the orange juice to the cooked or canned apricots. Cool a little, then purée in a liquidiser. Divide this between 4 or 6 stemmed, wide glasses (or coupes).

■ For the topping, purée the cheese with the remaining orange juice and the yogurt. Spoon over the apricot purée and scatter with the almonds. Chill before serving.

4 SERVINGS		6 SERVINGS	
kcals	155	kcals	105
kJ	655	kJ	440
CHO	25 g	CHO	20 g
Fibre	14 g	Fibre	9 g

VARIATION

THIS RECIPE WORKS VERY WELL with many fresh stoned fruits, such as peaches or plums as well as with soft fruits like strawberries, raspberries, loganberries or mulberries. Of course, fresh fruit will not need soaking but, if using the soft fruits, it is advisable to sieve them after cooking (they need only 5 minutes simmering) to remove the small pips.

Almond Tart

A DELICIOUS TART which can be served as a pudding or cut into slices for afternoon tea. It keeps extremely well in an airtight tin and can also be frozen.

INGREDIENTS

175 g (6 oz) wholemeal shortcrust pastry (see page 126), with 2–3 drops of almond essence added

For the filling

100 g (4 oz) dried apricots or dried peaches, soaked overnight or 60 ml (4 tbsp) diabetic apricot jam

50 g (2 oz) butter or polyunsaturated margarine

2 eggs, size 2, beaten

50 g (2 oz) wholemeal self-raising flour

75 g (3 oz) ground almonds

2–3 drops almond essence

45–60 ml (3–4 tbsp) freshly squeezed orange juice

15 g (½ oz) flaked almonds

SERVES 8

■ Put the apricots in a pan with 300 ml (½ pint) of the soaking water and cook gently until soft. Purée and leave to cool.

■ Make the pastry, then roll out and use to line a lightly oiled 20 cm (8 inch) flan dish. Prick the base with a thin-pronged fork. Chill until needed.

■ Soften the butter, without melting, then blend with the eggs in a bowl until frothy and light. Gradually add the flour, ground almonds, almond essence and enough orange juice to make a soft, dropping consistency.

■ Spread the apricot purée evenly over the base of the pastry case. Pour over the almond mixture, level the top and sprinkle with the flaked almonds. Bake at 190°C (375°F) mark 5 for 35–40 minutes or until firm to the touch.

8 SERVINGS	
kcals	390
kJ	1620
CHO	25 g
Fibre	8 g

Chocolate and Coffee Mousse

IF USING AN ALCOHOL in the mixture, it is a good idea to make the mousse the day before to allow the flavours time to merge.

INGREDIENTS
100 g (4 oz) diabetic dark chocolate
30 ml (2 tbsp) strong black coffee with 2.5 ml (½ tsp) fructose, or 15 ml (1 tbsp) black coffee and 15 ml (1 tbsp) brandy or rum
5 ml (1 tsp) butter
4 eggs, size 1, separated
15 ml (1 tbsp) flaked almonds
SERVES 4 – 6

■ Break the chocolate into pieces and put into a bowl with the sweetened coffee or coffee and brandy or rum mixture. Stand the bowl in a saucepan, containing 5 cm (2 inches) simmering water, large enough to take the bowl snugly with its top above the saucepan rim. Simmer gently, stirring with a wooden spoon, until the chocolate starts to melt. Remove from the heat and thoroughly blend with a wooden spoon until the melted chocolate has combined with the liquid. Never attempt to do this over direct heat or you will almost certainly end up with a flavour of burnt chocolate!

■ When the chocolate has cooled enough but still warm, add the butter, in small pieces, stirring with the wooden spoon until each piece is amalgamated; the chocolate mixture should then have the consistency of thick cream and a glossy appearance (due to the butter).

■ Stir in the egg yolks, one at a time, making sure that the mixture is quite smooth before the next is added. Whisk the egg whites until stiff and fold them gently but thoroughly into the mixture until no white spots are to be seen.

■ Put the chocolate mousse into individual stemmed, wide glasses (coupes) or into a glass bowl and scatter over the flaked almonds. Chill, but remove from the refrigerator 20 minutes before serving.

4 SERVINGS		6 SERVINGS	
kcals	235	kcals	160
kJ	990	kJ	660
CHO	5 g	CHO	Negligible
Fibre	Negligible	Fibre	Negligible

Plum Nut Crumble

A COMFORTING, cold weather family pudding.

INGREDIENTS
450 g (1 lb) ripe plums, halved and stoned
2 medium eating apples, peeled, cored and sliced
60 ml (4 tbsp) pure unsweetened apple juice
squeeze of fresh lemon juice
1 cm ($\frac{1}{2}$ inch) stick cinnamon
For the crumble topping
75 g (3 oz) wholemeal flour
50 g (2 oz) unsweetened muesli or rolled oats
15 g ($\frac{1}{2}$ oz) grated desiccated coconut
pinch of ground mixed spice
40 g (1$\frac{1}{2}$ oz) polyunsaturated margarine, melted
15 g ($\frac{1}{2}$ oz) flaked almonds or chopped walnuts
SERVES 4 – 6

▌Cook the plums and apples with the apple juice, lemon juice and cinnamon until soft. Transfer to an ovenproof dish, removing the stick cinnamon.

▌For the crumble, mix the dry ingredients together in a bowl. Add the melted margarine and mix quickly and thoroughly until none of the crumble remains dry. Sprinkle this evenly over the fruit and scatter the nuts on top.

▌Bake at 190°C (375°F) mark 5 for about 30 minutes until the top is crisp. Serve warm, with a little cream or yogurt.

4 SERVINGS		6 SERVINGS	
kcals	290	kcals	195
kJ	1215	kJ	815
CHO	40 g	CHO	25 g
Fibre	7 g	Fibre	5 g

VARIATIONS

MANY DIFFERENT FRUITS in season, such as blackberries, blueberries or gooseberries, are also good served this way, with or without apple.

Other unsweetened fruit juices can be used according to your inclination.

When fresh fruit is scarce, soaked dried fruits, such as apricots, peaches, pears and prunes, can be used, either individually or in combination.

Curd Tart

THIS COOKED CURD CAKE is, I think, the most delicious of all cheesecake recipes. If wished, put cooked or raw fruit on the top of the soft, creamy filling. However, in its simple form this cheesecake is really excellent.

INGREDIENTS
150 g (5 oz) wholemeal shortcrust pastry, chilled (see page 126)
For the filling
275 g (10 oz) curd cheese, drained, cottage cheese, sieved, or quark
30 ml (2 tbsp) ground almonds
75 g (3 oz) sultanas
finely grated rind of 1 lemon
juice of $\frac{1}{2}$ lemon
15 g ($\frac{1}{2}$ oz) melted butter
2 eggs, size 1, separated
pinch of freshly grated nutmeg
SERVES 6

■ Roll out the pastry and use to line an oiled 18 cm (7 inch) flan dish. Chill.

■ For the filling, mix the curd cheese, ground almonds, lemon rind and juice and melted butter (which must not be allowed to brown) together in a bowl.

■ Beat the egg yolks and brush a little over the base of the pastry case, to prevent it from becoming soggy, and prick lightly. Mix the remaining egg yolk well into the cheese mixture. Whisk the egg whites until stiff and gently fold them into the filling. Spoon the mixture into the pastry case and sprinkle the top with the freshly grated nutmeg.

■ Bake at 190°C (375°F) mark 5 for 30–35 minutes or until risen and golden brown. Serve cold but not chilled, cut into wedges.

6 SERVINGS	
kcals	635
kJ	2665
CHO	45 g
Fibre	8 g

Gâteau des Crêpes

GÂTEAU DES CRÊPES is a favourite pancake pudding of mine. In selecting the fruit or fruits, the sweeter, less tart, fruits should be your choice. You will need 450 g (1 lb) fruit to make 300 ml (½ pint) cooked puréed fruit.

INGREDIENTS
four × 15–17 cm (6–7 inch) pancakes, warm (see page 134)
45 ml (3 tbsp) curd cheese, drained, or quark
300 ml (½ pint) fruit, cooked without liquid, puréed
30 ml (2 tbsp) natural yogurt, preferably Greek strained

SERVES 4 – 6

■ Place the first pancake on the base of a greased ovenproof dish, slightly larger in diameter than the pancakes. Spread 25 ml (1½ tbsp) of the curd cheese on top of the pancake and lay over another pancake. Cover this with a layer of the puréed fruit and the third pancake. Cover the third pancake with the remaining curd cheese and put the last pancake on top.

■ Mix the remaining fruit purée with the yogurt and pour over the pancakes. Heat through at 180°C (350°F) mark 4 for 20 minutes.

4 SERVINGS		6 SERVINGS	
kcals	360	kcals	240
kJ	1510	kJ	1005
CHO	40 g	CHO	25 g
Fibre	5.5 g	Fibre	4 g

VARIATIONS

IF YOU HAVE NOT TIME to prepare the fruit purée, fruit canned in its own juice, drained, may be puréed and used instead. If needed, add a little of the can juice to ensure that the purée is not too dry.

A jam with no added sugar instead of the fruit purée and soured or whipped double cream instead of the yogurt also make a good variation.

Pancakes

PANCAKES ARE A MOST USEFUL FOOD to have available. Interleaved with grease-proof paper, they will keep in the refrigerator for 4–5 days and for months in the freezer. They can be used with either sweet or savoury fillings. Wholemeal pancakes are deliciously nutty; think, for instance, of the Brittany crêpes and some of the Russian ones served with soured cream and caviare. It is always wise to make more than you need immediately, then either chill or freeze the remainder.

INGREDIENTS

175 g (6 oz) wholemeal plain flour

2.5 ml (½ tsp) salt

2 eggs, size 3, beaten

450 ml (¾ pint) skimmed milk or made-up powdered skimmed milk

15 ml (1 tbsp) sunflower oil or melted butter

few drops of ice cold water

small nut of butter or polyunsaturated margarine, for each pancake

MAKES TWELVE 15–17 cm (6–7 inch) PANCAKES

■ Put the flour and salt into a bowl and mix thoroughly. Make a 'well' in the centre and drop in the eggs. Stir briskly, turning in the flour from the edges of the bowl. Add half the milk and stir vigorously to produce a thick batter, then beat in the oil or butter and, lastly, the remainder of the milk. Whisk vigorously, turning the bowl periodically as you do so, until bubbles cover the surface. Leave to stand, covered with a cloth, at moderate room temperature, for a minimum of 30 minutes.

■ After standing, whisk again, adding the few drops of cold water. If possible, use a 18 cm (7 inch) non-stick pan. For the first pancake, melt a nut of butter, 2.5 cm (1 inch) across until foaming. Spread it evenly over the pan surface but do not allow it to brown. Spoon 30 ml (2 tbsp) of the batter into the centre of the pan and, tilting the pan in every direction, form it into a thin layer of even thickness all over the base of the pan. Shake the pan from time to time and, when the pancake begins to shift, you will know that the underside is dry and beginning to colour.

■ Flip it over, or turn with a non-stick slice, and inspect the pancake. When it is a speckled golden brown, it is done and you can cook the other side for the same amount of time. The thin outer edge should, by then, be slightly crisp.

■ If the pancakes are to be eaten at once, slide on to a warmed plate on a plate warmer or keep hot over a saucepan of hot water. Add another nut of butter to the pan and repeat the process. Only practice will give you the skill needed for this operation but a very few trials will soon give you the knack. By about the third pancake the stove may be becoming too hot, so be ready to reduce the heat. If you are using an electric hob, the response will be slower so you may have to allow the pan to cool a little in between, but it must not be allowed to become too cool or the pancake will turn out leathery and palid. If you are lucky enough to have a griddle, the cooking is rather easier as the heat can be more controlled and constant. Experience is the only way, but it is fun acquiring it. As they are cooked, stack the pancakes on top of one another on the warmed plate.

PER PANCAKE	
kcals	105
kJ	440
CHO	10 g
Fibre	1 g

Christmas Pudding

AN APPROVED FESTIVE PUDDING RECIPE which is excellent, enjoyed by diabetics and non-diabetics alike. It should be made at least 3 weeks before Christmas, to give time for the flavours to mature. This recipe freezes excellently and can be kept in the freezer, without loss of flavour, for a year if need be.

INGREDIENTS
75 g (3 oz) currants
75 g (3 oz) raisins
75 g (3 oz) sultanas
100 g (4 oz) wholemeal flour
100 g (4 oz) fresh wholemeal breadcrumbs
25 g (1 oz) blanched almonds, finely chopped
10 ml (2 tsp) ground mixed spice
pinch of salt
1 medium carrot, scraped and grated
finely grated rind and juice of 1 lemon
75 g (3 oz) polyunsaturated margarine, melted
3 eggs, size 4, beaten
150 ml ($\frac{1}{4}$ pint) Guinness' stout
SERVES 8

∎ Mix all the ingredients together in a large bowl, starting with the dry ones and adding the margarine, beaten eggs and stout last of all.

∎ Transfer the mixture to a lightly oiled 600 ml (1 pint) pudding basin, preferably one with a metal clip lid, leaving a space about 2 cm ($\frac{3}{4}$ inch) deep at the top for expansion. Cover with greased greaseproof paper tied around the rim, then with the clip lid or with a double thickness of foil well secured.

∎ Steam the pudding for $2\frac{1}{2}$–3 hours. When ready, remove the top coverings to let out the air. Do not be alarmed at the light colour of the top of the pudding, it will darken considerably during the second boiling on Christmas Day! Put on a new covering in the same way as the last and store, either in the refrigerator or the freezer.

∎ On the day of serving, steam again for 1 hour, turn out on to a warmed serving dish and decorate with the traditional sprig of holly. Serve with cream.

8 SERVINGS	
kcals	260
kJ	1090
CHO	35 g
Fibre	5 g

Spicy Carrot Cake

IN EARLY IRISH LITERATURE in a 9th century poem, wild carrots were referred to as 'honey underground...'. The cultivated variety certainly sweeten this delicious, spicy cake.

INGREDIENTS

150 g (5 oz) dried dates, stoned and finely chopped
100 ml (4 fl oz) water
175 g (6 oz) butter or polyunsaturated margarine, softened
2 eggs, size 2, beaten
225 g (8 oz) wholemeal self-raising flour
175 g (6 oz) carrot, scraped and finely grated
25 g (1 oz) ground almonds
finely grated rind of 1 large orange
2.5 ml (½ tsp) ground ginger
2.5 ml (½ tsp) ground cinnamon
2.5 ml (½ tsp) ground mixed spice
15–30 ml (1–2 tbsp) hazelnuts, chopped (optional)
For the icing and filling
two × 200 g (7 oz) tubs quark
25 g (1 oz) butter or polyunsaturated margarine, softened
finely grated rind of 1 large orange
ground cinnamon, for sprinkling

MAKES ABOUT 12 SLICES

▪ Simmer the dates in the water for about 10 minutes until soft, then stone and chop them finely. Blend the dates, the liquid in which they were cooked, the butter and eggs together until creamy. Gently, but very thoroughly, fold in the remaining ingredients, in the order given.

▪ Spoon the mixture into an oiled and lined 18 cm (7 inch) cake tin and level the top. Bake at 180°C (350°F) mark 4 for about 1 hour, testing with a skewer to make sure that the centre is cooked. Remove from the oven and allow to cool in the tin for 5 minutes before turning out on to a wire rack to cool completely. Remove the lining paper.

▪ Beat all the ingredients for the icing together and, if too stiff, add a little orange juice to make a spreading consistency. Carefully slice the cake in half horizontally and spread the filling to a depth of 1 cm (½ inch). Sandwich the cake and cover with the remainder of the icing. Sprinkle with ground cinnamon.

PER SLICE	
kcals	285
kJ	1190
CHO	20 g
Fibre	4 g

Nectarine and Orange Flan

A GOOD, light, fresh fruit flan, pleasant served warm or cold.

INGREDIENTS

175 g (6 oz) wholemeal shortcrust pastry, chilled (see page 126)
For the filling
3 ripe nectarines, halved and stoned
225 g (8 oz) curd cheese or quark
150 ml (¼ pint) freshly squeezed orange juice
2 eggs, size 1, beaten
5 ml (1 tsp) finely grated orange rind

SERVES ABOUT 6

- Roll out the pastry and use to line an oiled 20 cm (8 inch) flan dish. Lightly prick the base with a fork.
- Slice the nectarines and arrange, over-lapping one another, in decreasing circles in the pastry case.
- Blend the cheese, orange juice and eggs together until very smooth and creamy. Pour over the fruit evenly and scatter the top with the orange rind.
- Bake at 190°C (375°F) mark 5 for about 30–40 minutes or until lightly set. Leave to cool, but do not chill or freeze.

6 SERVINGS	
kcals	405
kJ	1695
CHO	45 g
Fibre	5 g

VARIATIONS

GOOSEBERRIES, seedless grapes, peeled and stoned peaches or pears, sprinkled with lemon juice can be used.

For a lighter flan, omit the curd cheese.

If calories are a real problem, prepare the dessert without the pastry case. Cook the fruit, prepared as above, in a greased ovenproof dish standing in a larger dish containing 2.5 cm (1 inch) water. Cook in the oven at the same temperature for about 30 minutes.

Carob Fruit Cake

THIS TEMPTING CAKE KEEPS WELL in an airtight tin and can also be frozen.

INGREDIENTS
450 g (1 lb) raisins
275 ml (10 fl oz) unsweetened orange juice
175 g (6 oz) butter or polyunsaturated margarine, softened
3 eggs, size 2, beaten
250 g (9 oz) wholemeal flour
75 g (3 oz) carob flour or powder
10 ml (2 tsp) baking powder
finely grated rind of 2 oranges
25 g (1 oz) walnuts, chopped
MAKES ABOUT 12 SLICES

- Soak the raisins in the orange juice overnight.
- The next day, blend the butter and eggs together in a bowl until smooth. In an-other bowl, thoroughly mix the flours and baking powder. Gradually add the egg and butter mixture, then the raisins, orange juice and rind. Lastly, add the walnuts, mixing gently but thoroughly.
- Spoon the mixture into an oiled and lined 18 cm (7 inch) cake tin and level the top. Bake at 180°C (350°F) mark 4 for 1 hour. Reduce the oven temperature to 170°C (325°F) mark 3 and bake for a further 45 minutes, testing with a skewer to ensure that the centre is cooked.
- Leave the cake in the tin for 15 minutes to firm, then put on to a wire rack.

PER SLICE	
kcals	325
kJ	1350
CHO	45 g
Fibre	5 g

Fruit Cake

THIS IS EXCELLENT FOR WEDDINGS, birthdays, Christmas or other celebrations. The recipe works just as well with the quantities of the ingredients doubled. Recipes for diabetic marzipan and icing follow.

INGREDIENTS

50 g (2 oz) butter or polyunsaturated margarine
25 g (1 oz) fructose
75 g (3 oz) sultanas
75 g (3 oz) raisins
75 g (3 oz) currants
3 dried apricots, soaked for at least 4 hours, finely chopped
225 ml (8 fl oz) Guinness' stout
225 g (8 oz) wholemeal self-raising flour
5 ml (1 tsp) instant coffee powder
7.5 ml (1½ tsp) ground mixed spice
75 g (3 oz) walnuts, chopped
3 eggs, size 3, beaten
30 ml (2 tbsp) brandy, rum or whisky

MAKES 14 SLICES

■ Bring the butter, fructose, dried fruit and stout to the boil in a saucepan and simmer for 20 minutes. Leave to cool.

■ Mix together the flour, coffee powder, spice and walnuts in a bowl. Add the eggs and the fruit and stout mixture. Mix gently but thoroughly, finally pouring in 15 ml (1 tbsp) of the spirit and mixing again.

■ Spoon the mixture into an oiled and lined 20 cm (8 inch) cake tin and level the top leaving a slight depression in the centre. Bake on the shelf below the centre of the oven at 180°C (350°F) mark 4 for 20 minutes. Lower the oven temperature to 150°C (300°F) mark 2 and bake for a further 1–1½ hours, covering the top with greaseproof paper if becoming too brown. Test with a skewer to make sure the centre is cooked. Cool in the tin for 15 minutes before turning out on to a wire rack to cool completely. Remove the lining paper.

■ When quite cold, carefully turn the cake upside down and, with a very thin skewer or cocktail stick, make a number of holes penetrating to the centre on the bottom. With a small spoon, gently pour the remainder of the spirit into these holes. Wrap in greaseproof paper and store in an airtight tin. It freezes very well for 6 months.

PER SLICE

kcals	185
kJ	770
CHO	20 g
Fibre	3 g

Diabetic Marzipan

THIS RECIPE IS FROM the British Diabetic Association.

INGREDIENTS

100 g (4 oz) ground almonds
50 g (2 oz) fructose
25 g (1 oz) cornflour
1 egg, size 1, beaten
15 ml (1 tbsp) diabetic apricot jam, warmed

SUFFICIENT TO COAT THE TOP AND SIDES OF THE FRUIT CAKE ABOVE

■ Beat the ground almonds, fructose, cornflour and egg together until the mixture is a smooth paste, using the fingers if necessary. Divide into 2 equal portions.

■ Scatter a little cornflour on to a work surface and roll out and shape one portion of marzipan to fit the base of the cake. Cut the top of the cake level with a knife and turn it upside down; from now on the bottom of the cake will be the top. Paint this surface with the warm jam, invert it once more and press it down on to the round of marzipan.

■ While the jam is cooling and sticking the marzipan round to the cake, roll out and shape the other portion of marzipan to form a strip that will go exactly around the side of the cake. When it is ready and has been tried for a fit, paint the side of the cake with the warm jam and apply the strip of marzipan, pressing evenly around and smoothing over the join. A strip of cloth, wound around the outside of the marzipan strip and secured, will hold it in place until the jam has cooled and set.

■ When the jam has set, the cake can be inverted again, the cloth strip removed and the circular join between the top and the side marzipan can be smoothed over. Do not freeze this marzipan.

TOTAL	
kcals	960
kJ	4015
CHO	25 g
Fibre	15 g

Diabetic Icing

IF POSSIBLE, do not prepare this icing until the day on which the cake is to be eaten. This recipe is from the British Diabetic Association.

INGREDIENTS
50 g (2 oz) fructose
pinch of salt
1 egg white
2.5 ml ($\frac{1}{2}$ tsp) lemon juice

SUFFICIENT TO ICE THE FRUIT CAKE GIVEN ON PAGE 138

■ Put the fructose into a liquidiser or food processor and blend until the powder becomes as fine as ordinary icing sugar. Transfer to a bowl and mix in the salt well. Whisk in the egg white and lemon juice.

■ Transfer the bowl to a saucepan a quarter full of simmering water and continue whisking until stiff peaks form. Take from the heat and continue whisking until cool. Spread over the marzipan on the cake with a spatula.

TOTAL	
kcals	205
kJ	850
CHO	Negligible
Fibre	0

PRESERVES

IN GENERAL, sweet preserves should be regarded as almost forbidden fruit, except in small quantities. All can be made with fructose but, as it has the same calorific value as other sugars, such preserves are not suitable for those with a weight problem. From a CHO point of view, 5 ml (1 tsp) jam or marmalade made with fructose is counted as between 1–2 g CHO according to the fruit used and can be regarded as negligible in the daily CHO intake.

Unfortunately, compared with the price of ordinary sugar, fructose is unreasonably expensive and 450 g (1 lb) jam or jelly made with it can be a luxury for many. There are, now, some extremely good jams made without added sugar but, once opened, they must be kept in a refrigerator and used up fairly rapidly or they will go mouldy. If you cannot find your favourite variety, follow the recipe in any good preserve book, using fructose instead of sugar, but do not take heed of those who say that you only need half the quantity, compared to sugar, because fructose is twice as sweet. It is perfectly true that it is so, but your jam will neither set properly nor keep well if you do not use the same amount of fructose as sugar. Remember, however, all jams made with fructose, in this way, must be regarded as restricted items and taken fully into consideration in planning your diet balance.

All the preserves I have made in this way keep perfectly, although I still recommend you to keep them in a refrigerator once opened. Be quite certain too that the glass jars you are using are perfectly clean, dry and have been properly sterilised, either by microwaving them at **5** for 5 minutes, or heating them in a very slow oven for 20 minutes. If using plastic lined, screw-on tops (my favourite—many products come in these today, so they are worth keeping), these must be sterilised as being metal, you cannot put them into the microwave oven. Put them in a saucepan containing just enough boiling water to cover. Boil, covered, for 6 minutes. Strain off the water and put the saucepan lid on again until you are ready to fill the jars. Leave the jars in the oven until just before you are going to fill them and, if sterilising in the microwave oven, do this just before you need them. In either case, they will be hot and you will need a cloth to handle them. Do not allow the cloth to come into contact with the upper part of the rim or the inside of the jars. Hold them by the outside, with the cloth, to keep the inside sterile. This may seem a lot of fuss, but the keeping quality of your preserves really does depend on good sterilisation.

A sugar thermometer is most useful to assist you in obtaining a really good setting. Start with slightly under-ripe fruit, high in pectin, such as apple, black, red and white currants, cranberries, plums and raspberries. Blackberries, which have less pectin, should have some apple added to them. Add 15 ml (1 tbsp) lemon juice to every 450 g (1 lb) fruit low in pectin, such as strawberries, cherries, pears and peaches.

Having said this, I will only add that, in my experience no commercial product can compete in taste with the home-made preserves. This is most noticeably so in the case of the thick-cut marmalades, which is why I make a year's supply every January, when the Seville oranges arrive, with the recipe on page 142.

I have never seen commercially made diabetic chutneys on sale, but it is very easy to make your own. Some need no added sweetening at all and others, only a little. Using 5 ml (1 tsp) of any of the chutneys has a negligible CHO value, but it is not wise to eat them too lavishly. As you know, a little is delicious with cheese, cold meats or poultry. A teaspoonful is excellent mixed into a casserole or a minced beef dish and, of course, accompanying a curry.

Thick-cut Dundee Marmalade

THIS DELICIOUS HOME-MADE PRESERVE is well worth the trouble as it will last the year through. Seville oranges are available in January and February.

INGREDIENTS
2.3 kg (5 lb) fructose
1.4 kg (3 lb) Seville oranges, slightly under-ripe
1.7 litres (3 pints) water
2 lemons
MAKES ABOUT 2.3 kg (8 lb)

■ Open the fructose and put in a warm dry place, such as the top of the stove, to dry off any moisture.

■ Wash the oranges well, dry them and pick off any stalks. Put them, whole, into a large saucepan with 1.4 litres (2½ pints) of the water. Bring to the boil, cover and simmer gently for about 1 hour or until the peel is soft enough to squeeze between the fingers. This is important, as once fructose is added the peel will soften no more.

■ When the peel of the oranges is soft, take the saucepan off the heat and, taking out 2 or 3 oranges at a time, put them on a large meat dish and slice them in half. Scoop the interior flesh out with a large dessertspoon and put it, pips and all, into a medium saucepan, stacking and reserving the empty skins. Continue until all the oranges are halved, scooped out and the pulp and pips transferred to the other saucepan.

■ Squeeze the lemons and add the juice to the liquid in the large saucepan and the peels to the orange pulp in the medium one. Cover the pulp with the remaining 300 ml (½ pint) water and bring the medium saucepan to the boil and simmer for 20 minutes.

■ Meanwhile, with a half-moon chopper or a sharp knife, chop the orange peel into the sized chunks you prefer. When the medium pan has simmered for 20 minutes, strain the juice from it into the liquid in the large saucepan, pressing the pulp to extract the last of the pectin. If you have a couple of chinois sieves (conical strainers), one larger than the other, put a quantity of the pulp into the larger and press the smaller into it, which gives a very efficient extraction.

■ When you have finished chopping the peel, return it all to the liquid in the large saucepan and stir in the fructose well with a wooden spoon. **Now comes the most important part**. Once the fructose is added, the marmalade must be heated over a moderate heat and **stirred continually without being allowed to come to the boil until every grain of the fructose is dissolved**. If the marmalade is allowed to boil before this happens, it is almost certain to crystallise and spoil. In stirring, wash down any grains of fructose that have stuck to the sides of the saucepan, which is why it is worth while to pour the powdered fructose into the middle of the liquid, when adding.

■ When you are really satisfied, by scraping the bottom and corners, that every grain is gone, bring to the boil rapidly and maintain as high a boiling as will be possible without the saucepan boiling over— **this needs watching**. If using, clip your sugar thermometer to the side of the saucepan, making sure that its end is at least

2.5 cm (1 inch) beneath the surface of the liquid (not just the foam on top). For the quantities given, the setting point should be reached in about 20–25 minutes, but this depends on the amount of pectin in the fruit. If you do not have a sugar thermometer, take out a spoonful of the **liquid** (not the foam) and pour it on to a cold saucer. If wrinkles form as it cools and it sets in a light jelly, the marmalade is done, which should co-incide with a sugar thermometer temperature of 110°C (225°F). Continue boiling at the same rate for a further 5 minutes, then take off the heat. On no account continue boiling if the marmalade begins to darken noticeably in colour or its flavour will be spoiled, better a soft marmalade, if your fruit is deficient in pectin, than a ruined batch.

▌ Allow the marmalade to stand, covered, for 5 minutes, then bottle in the sterilised glass jars. This will ensure that all the peel does not float up to the top. A sterilised wide-mouthed funnel and a ladle are useful in avoiding messy drips. When the jars are full, seal at once with the sterilised lids.

PER 25 g (1 oz)		TOTAL	
kcals	70	kcals	9130
kJ	300	kJ	38,200
CHO	Negligible	CHO	120 g
Fibre	Negligible	Fibre	35 g

VARIATIONS

AS WELL AS SEVILLE ORANGES, marmalade can be made with sweet oranges (though the fragrance is not as fine), grapefruit, lemons or limes or a mixture of fruits.

Lemon Mincemeat

THIS HAS A LOVELY, fresh, uncloying taste which offsets other rich Christmas foods. Do not make this mincemeat earlier than the beginning of December, unless you intend to freeze it.

INGREDIENTS
4 lemons, washed
225 g (8 oz) sultanas
75 g (3 oz) dried dates, stoned and finely chopped
75 g (3 oz) raisins
3 sweet eating apples, such as Cox's Orange Pippins, peeled, cored and finely chopped
1 medium carrot, scraped and finely chopped
50 g (2 oz) candied peel, chopped, rinsed in warm water to desugar
75 g (3 oz) blanched almonds, finely chopped
10 ml (2 tsp) ground mixed spice
25 g (1 oz) fructose
60 ml (4 tbsp) brandy, whisky or dry sherry
MAKES 700 g (1½ lb)

▌ Squeeze the juice from the lemons and reserve. Cut the rind into strips and boil in water to cover for 5 minutes, then throw away the water and repeat the process; this will remove any bitterness from the lemon rind. Drain the strips, removing any of the softened white pith, and finely chop the remaining rind.

▌ In a bowl, mix the lemon juice with all the other ingredients, except the spirit. Lastly, add two-thirds of the spirit.

▌ Put the mincemeat into clean, sterilised jars (see page 141), adding a little of the remaining spirit to cover the mincemeat. Seal the jars and store in a cool place or in the refrigerator.

PER 25 g (1 oz)	
kcals	45
kJ	190
CHO	10 g
Fibre	1 g

VARIATION

IF MAKING A LARGE MINCEMEAT FLAN, make a first layer of cooked, puréed apple flavoured with lemon juice with a layer of mincemeat on top, the effect is far finer than with mincemeat alone.

Brandied Peaches, Nectarines or Apricots

A DELICIOUS PRESERVE at any time of the year; costly to buy but far cheaper to make. Especially if using peaches, care must be taken to carry the preparation out rapidly or they will discolour. Wide-necked bottling jars are essential.

INGREDIENTS

1 kg (2¼ lb) peaches, apricots or nectarines

600 ml (1 pint) salted water, using 5 ml (1 tsp) salt, dissolved

100 g (4 oz) fructose

300 ml (½ pint) water

90 ml (6 tbsp) brandy

FILLS ABOUT THREE 450 g (1 lb) JARS, SERVES 4 PER JAR

■ To skin peaches or apricots, immerse in boiling water for 1 minute, then skin; the skin comes off easily without any loss of flesh. Nectarines do not need to be skinned. Halve each fruit by cutting along the natural groove running around it. Remove the stone and, at once, submerge each fruit under the salted water to prevent discolouration.

■ Dissolve the fructose in the plain water in a saucepan. Bring to the boil and boil, covered, for 2 minutes. Cool slightly and add the brandy, stirring to mix.

■ Rinse the fruit halves in warm water and put into sterilised jars (see page 141), making sure that no fruit projects into the neck of the jar. Cover at once with the brandied syrup and seal with a sterilised lid. Store in a cool, dark place for at least 1 month before using.

4 SERVINGS PER JAR	
kcals	75
kJ	310
CHO	5 g
Fibre	1 g

VARIATIONS

OTHER FRUIT SUCH AS stoned and pricked cherries, peeled and cored pears, or stoned plums, can also be preserved in this way.

For spiced fruit, omit the brandy and use the same amount of white wine vinegar in the syrup instead, as well as a 2.5 cm (1 inch) cinnamon stick, a few allspice berries, a few cloves and a blade of mace. Spicing is best with a fruit such as pears, plums or thick, unpeeled, orange slices. Spiced fruit is delicious with cold meats or poultry or as an addition to a mixed hors d'oeuvres.

Orange Chutney

A PIQUANT CHUTNEY to serve with cold meats, cheese and any cold meals.

INGREDIENTS

6 medium thin-skinned oranges, peeled
225 g (8 oz) onions, skinned and chopped
450 g (1 lb) dried dates, stoned and chopped
600 ml (1 pint) white malt vinegar
10 ml (2 tsp) ground ginger
10 ml (2 tsp) salt
MAKES ABOUT 1.8 kg (4 lb)

▮ Divide the oranges into segments, removing as much of the remaining pith as possible. Slit the segments, remove and discard any pips, then chop the segments very finely on a large dish. Alternatively, process in a food processor for 30 seconds.

▮ Transfer the orange to a large saucepan. Add the onions, dates, vinegar, ginger and salt, and mix well. Bring to the boil and simmer quite briskly for 1–1½ hours until golden brown and thick.

▮ Put the chutney into hot, sterilised jars. Seal at once with sterilised screw caps. These caps must be lined entirely with nylon on the inside, as chutneys are very corrosive to bare metal.

PER 25 g (1 oz)	
kcals	20
kJ	90
CHO	5 g
Fibre	1 g

VARIATIONS

USE 450 g (1 lb) DRIED APRICOTS, soaked for at least 4 hours in water barely to cover, instead of oranges. If you are using the soaking liquid, reduce the vinegar slightly.

Try 900 g (2 lb) peeled bananas instead of oranges.

Onion Chutney

AN INDIAN, uncooked chutney, which is excellent with a great many curries. It must be consumed within 2 days and is best kept in the refrigerator. Though not traditional, tarragon vinegar lends fragrance to this chutney.

INGREDIENTS

2 large mild Spanish onions, skinned and chopped
3 medium or 2 large tomatoes, skinned and chopped
salt to taste
1.25 ml (¼ tsp) cayenne pepper
15 ml (1 tbsp) white wine vinegar or tarragon vinegar
15 ml (1 tbsp) freshly squeezed lemon juice
SERVES 4

▮ Combine the onion and tomato in a bowl and add salt to taste. Scatter the cayenne pepper over and mix in thoroughly.

▮ Mix the vinegar and lemon juice together and pour over the chutney. Stir well. Transfer to a serving dish and chill.

4 SERVINGS	
kcals	35
kJ	145
CHO	10 g
Fibre	3 g

Apple Chutney

A GOOD WAY OF using up sound windfalls.

INGREDIENTS

1.4 kg (3 lb) cooking apples, peeled, cored and chopped
600 ml (1 pint) white malt vinegar
50 g (2 oz) fructose
10 ml (2 tsp) salt
10 ml (2 tsp) ground ginger
5 ml (1 tsp) dry English mustard powder (not whole-grain kind)
2.5 ml ($\frac{1}{2}$ tsp) cayenne pepper
100 g (4 oz) dried dates, stoned and chopped
100 g (4 oz) sultanas
225 g (8 oz) onions, skinned and chopped

MAKES ABOUT 1.8 kg (4 lb)

▌ Put the apples into lightly salted water to prevent discoloration. Put the vinegar, fructose, salt, ginger, mustard and pepper into a large saucepan and bring to the boil.

▌ Drain the apples and add to the pan with all the other ingredients. Bring again to the boil and simmer, uncovered, for 1–1½ hours until golden brown and thick. The apples will release juice, so continue boiling until the chutney is no longer runny.

▌ Pour the chutney into hot, sterilised jars and seal at once with sterilised nylon-lined lids.

PER 25 g (1 oz)	
kcals	15
kJ	65
CHO	5 g
Fibre	1 g

VARIATIONS

GOOSEBERRIES CAN BE USED with or without apples.

A mixture of 700 g (1½ lb) apples with the same amount of peeled, deseeded, sliced marrow makes a particularly appetising chutney. Add 15 ml (1 tbsp) ground turmeric during cooking, which will also help to thicken as well as give the chutney a fine colour and flavour.

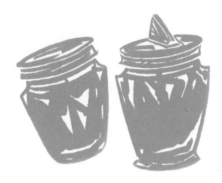

Red or Green Tomato Chutney

PERHAPS THE MOST POPULAR of all chutneys, with many uses. I am always undecided as to whether to skin the tomatoes or not. If green, leave the skin on, but if the tomatoes are ripe (when they are sweeter) some varieties can have rather tough skins. The skins provide a certain amount of roughage which is good in our diet. However, if you really dislike them in a chutney, stand the tomatoes in boiling water for 30 seconds and they can then easily be skinned. If liked, a mixture of red and green tomatoes can be used.

INGREDIENTS

1.4 kg (3 lb) tomatoes, red, green or mixed, coarsely chopped
450 g (1 lb) onions, skinned and finely chopped
1 celery heart, trimmed and finely chopped, or 3 large lovage leaves, finely chopped
300 ml ($\frac{1}{2}$ pint) white malt vinegar
2.5 ml ($\frac{1}{2}$ tsp) ground ginger
2.5 ml ($\frac{1}{2}$ tsp) ground cinnamon
1.25 ml ($\frac{1}{4}$ tsp) freshly grated nutmeg
10 ml (2 tsp) salt
5 ml (1 tsp) cayenne pepper
2–3 medium cooking apples, peeled, cored and chopped
150 g (5 oz) sultanas
50 g (2 oz) fructose (optional)

MAKES ABOUT 1.8 kg (4 lb)

■ Put the tomatoes into a large saucepan with the onions and celery. Add the vinegar, spices and seasoning. Bring to the boil and simmer, uncovered, for 1 hour.

■ Add the apples, sultanas and fructose, if using, but make sure it has completely dissolved before the chutney reaches boiling point again. Simmer quite briskly for 1–1½ hours or until the chutney is sufficiently reduced and thick. If very ripe tomatoes are used, they will produce a lot of juice which will take longer to boil down.

■ Put the chutney into hot, sterilised glass jars and seal at once with sterilised screw caps entirely lined with nylon.

PER 25 g (1 oz)	
kcals	15
kJ	65
CHO	5 g
Fibre	1 g

Chilli Sherry Relish

THIS EXCELLENT RELISH was brought from the West Indies nearly two hundred years ago. It gives a delicious fillip to consommé, eggs, fish, seafood, cheese dishes or grills. Only a few drops are needed, as with other hot chilli sauces, but this one is a little milder than most, being zesty rather than really hot.

INGREDIENTS

24 small dried chillies
12 allspice berries
6 whole cloves
750 ml (1¼ pints) dry sherry

MAKES 750 ml (1¼ pints)

■ Put all the dry ingredients into a wide-mouthed 900 ml (1½ pint) glass jar with a sealing screw-top. Fill up with the sherry. Screw down the cap securely and give several good shakes, inverting the jar a number of times.

■ Put the jar into a dark, cool place. Repeat the shaking twice a week for 6 weeks.

■ Transfer some of the relish into a smaller, dropping bottle, making sure that the spices remain in the large one. As the large jar becomes half full, it can be topped up with more sherry. This can be repeated 2 or 3 times before more spices are needed.

TOTAL	
kcals	915
kJ	3830
CHO	20 g
Fibre	0

LOW CALORIE
ALCOHOLIC DRINKS

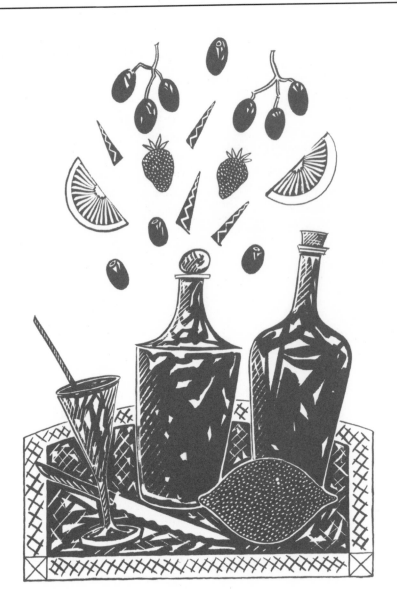

WITH THE EXCEPTION OF the sweet liqueurs and some sweetened whiskys, rums and, of course, sweet sherries, aperitifs and port, which should be used sparingly by all diabetics, most alcoholic drinks have a negligible CHO (carbohydrate) value. However, because alcohol is a carbohydrate sparer, it poses a problem for overweight diabetics or, incautiously used, even for those who have attained a good balance. The key to the whole business is, if you are seriously overweight, try to keep off alcohol completely. There are now a number of non-alcoholic, low calorie wines and beers available to help you do this, which are well worth finding out about. When you are back to normal weight, use alcohol with discretion.

For those of normal weight, 'moderation' is the operative word. There is no reason why you should not have the reasonable amounts of dry wines and beers that make a meal more enjoyable and appetising. When taken in moderation with food, alcohol disturbs a diabetic's balance far less than if it is taken alone. In fact, all alcoholic drinks served at parties where diabetics are present should be accompanied by some source of CHO, even if it is only a well planned plate of canapés or dips with toast or biscuits. Beware of some of the vegetable dips which may have hardly any CHO value at all! If in doubt, don't be in the least shy in asking for some bread or toast.

Buck's Fizz

THE PRINCE OF PRE-MEAL DRINKS, it is simplicity itself and can be made using other Champagne-method dry, sparkling white wines.

INGREDIENTS
75 ml (2½ fl oz) fresh natural orange juice, chilled
75 ml (2½ fl oz) dry NV Champagne or other dry, sparkling white wine, chilled
SERVES 1

■ Pour the chilled orange juice into a Paris goblet. Gently top up with the Champagne.

1 SERVING	
kcals	80
kJ	335
CHO	10 g
Fibre	0

DRY SHERRY IS ALSO GOOD served in this way or a dry still wine or dry Italian or French vermouth. These drinks can all be pre-mixed and chilled, but, of course, any sparkling wine must be opened and drunk at once.

Sangria

THIS SPANISH RED WINE PUNCH is most useful for parties. It should be noted that some recipes for Sangria are sweetened, so do enquire if necessary.

INGREDIENTS
2 bottles of dry red wine, chilled
freshly squeezed juice of 2 lemons
1 double measure of brandy
washed peel of 1 cucumber, cut into large strips
2 peaches, stoned, skinned and cut into slices
MAKES 16–20 GLASSES

■ Combine all the ingredients in a punch bowl. Leave at moderate room temperature for 2 hours before serving.

16 SERVINGS		20 SERVINGS	
kcals	75	kcals	60
kJ	315	kJ	250
CHO	Negligible	CHO	Negligible
Fibre	Negligible	Fibre	Negligible

INSTEAD OF PEACHES, use the same amount of whatever fruit is in season.

Pineapple Julep

A DELICIOUS DRINK for a number of people, which comes from the Southern States of the United States of America. Do not make this drink earlier than 1 hour before serving.

INGREDIENTS

crushed ice

freshly squeezed juice of 2 oranges

150 ml ($\frac{1}{4}$ pint) gin, vodka or dry pale rum

1 small, ripe, pineapple, peeled, cored and chopped, or 175 g (6 oz) can of pineapple chunks in natural juice

75 dl bottle of dry, sparkling Moselle or dry sparkling wine

few sprigs of mint, burnet or borage, to decorate

SERVES 6

■ Fill a 1.1 litre (2 pint) jug a quarter full with crushed ice, add the orange juice and gin or other spirit, stirring well. Add the pineapple and finally the sparkling white wine, stir very gently and chill.

■ Just before serving, decorate with a few fragrant herb leaves. (If using canned unsweetened pineapple, in its natural juice, add a little of this, cautiously, until the drink tastes right.)

6 SERVINGS	
kcals	160
kJ	665
CHO	5 g
Fibre	0

White Wine Cup

ANOTHER GOOD PARTY DRINK with a fruit juice basis. Do not make this drink longer than 1 hour before serving.

INGREDIENTS

1 litre packet or can of unsweetened orange juice, chilled

1 litre packet or can of unsweetened grapefruit or pineapple juice, chilled

freshly squeezed juice of 2 lemons

3 bottles of dry white wine, chilled

$\frac{1}{2}$ bottle of gin or vodka, chilled

12 drops of Chilli sherry relish (see page 147) or 12 drops of Angostura Bitters

1 litre soda water, chilled

mint leaves or $\frac{1}{2}$ cucumber, sliced

2 trays of ice cubes

MAKES ABOUT 40 GLASSES

■ Mix together all the ingredients except the ice cubes in a large punch bowl. Keep chilled, if possible, and add the ice cubes only at the last moment. If the refrigerator is not large enough to take the punch bowl, distribute the punch between several jugs.

40 SERVINGS	
kcals	75
kJ	315
CHO	5 g
Fibre	0

VARIATION

IF SERVING AT THE HEIGHT OF THE SUMMER, a few sliced fruits can be used but do not make it appear like a fruit salad!

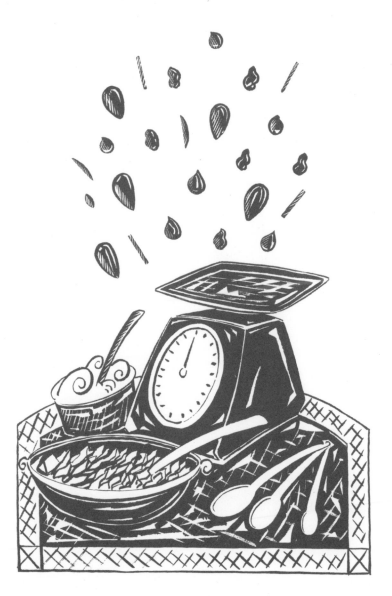

IT IS VERY IMPORTANT that diabetics follow the diet they have been prescribed as part of their medical treatment.

This list shows:

(a) foods that provide 10 grams carbohydrate (equivalent to 1 exchange, 1 portion, 1 unit or 1 line) when eaten in the quantities stated;

(b) foods that contain negligible amounts of carbohydrate, but appreciable amounts of energy (calories and kilojoules) which should be taken into account by those trying to lose weight.

Quantities are given in both 'spoon' measures as well as weights in grams and ounces. The tablespoon (tbsp) is based on a LEVEL 15 ml spoon, and the teaspoon (tsp) on a LEVEL 5 ml spoon.

It is recommended that a least half your daily energy should come from unrefined carbohydrates. The foods printed with an asterisk * are good sources of fibre.

151

BREAD

Choose *wholemeal or *wholewheat bread instead of white or brown whenever possible.

If using unsliced bread remember that:

▌ *Wholemeal/*wholewheat bread contains approximately 10 g CHO and 50 kcals/210 kJ in every 25 g/oz.

▌ White bread contains approximately 15 g CHO and 65 kcals/270 kJ in every 25 g/oz.

▌ Figures for carbohydrate and kcals are printed on the packaging of many sliced breads.

BREAKFAST CEREALS	Approximate measure	Approximate weight of food in g/oz containing 10 g CHO	kcals/kJ content
* Allbran	75 ml/5 tbsp	20 g/⅔ oz	50/210
* Bran Buds	60 ml/4 tbsp	20 g/⅔ oz	50/210
Cornflakes	75 ml/5 tbsp	10 g/⅓ oz	40/165
* Muesli (unsweetened)	30 ml/2 tbsp	15 g/½ oz	50/210
Muesli (sweetened)	30 ml/2 tbsp	15 g/½ oz	55/230
* Porridge (made with water)	60 ml/4 tbsp	120 g/4 oz	55/230
* Puffed Wheat	225 ml/15 tbsp	15 g/½ oz	50/210
Rice Krispies	180 ml/6 tbsp	10 g/⅓ oz	40/165
* Shredded Wheat	⅔ of one	—	50/210
Special K	120 ml/8 tbsp	15 g/½ oz	50/210
* Weetabix	1	—	60/250
* Weetaflakes	60 ml/4 tbsp	15 g/½ oz	50/210

OTHER CEREALS	Approximate measure	Approximate weight of food in g/oz containing 10 g CHO	kcals/kJ content
Arrowroot/Custard Powder/Cornflour	15 ml/1 tbsp	10 g/⅓ oz	35/145
Barley, raw	15 ml/1 tbsp	10 g/⅓ oz	40/165
Flour, plain, white	22 ml/1½ tbsp	10 g/⅓ oz	40/165
Flour, self-raising, white	22 ml/1½ tbsp	10 g/⅓ oz	45/190
* Flour, wholemeal/wholewheat	30 ml/2 tbsp	15 g/½ oz	50/210
* Oats, uncooked	45 ml/3 tbsp	15 g/½ oz	60/250
Rice, white, uncooked	15 ml/1 tbsp	10 g/⅓ oz	45/190
* Rice, brown, uncooked	15 ml/1 tbsp	10 g/⅓ oz	40/165
Spaghetti, white, uncooked	6 long (48 cm/ 19 inch) strands	10 g/⅓ oz	45/190
* Spaghetti, wholewheat, uncooked	20 short (25 cm/ 10 inch) strands	15 g/½ oz	50/210
Sago/Tapioca/Semolina, uncooked	10 ml/2 tsp	10 g/⅓ oz	35/145
* Soya flour, full fat	210 ml/14 tbsp	75 g/3 oz	300/1255
* Soya flour, low fat	135 ml/9 tbsp	50 g/2 oz	125/525
* Soya granules, dry	195 ml/13 tbsp	75 g/3 oz	200/835

* High fibre

BISCUITS/CRACKERS/ CRISPBREADS	Approximate measure	Approximate weight of food in g/oz containing 10 g CHO	kcals/kJ content
Biscuits, plain	2	15 g/½ oz	60/250
* Biscuits, digestive or wholemeal	1	15 g/½ oz	70/290
Biscuits, cream or chocolate	1	10 g/⅓ oz	60/250
Crackers, plain	2	15 g/½ oz	70/290
Crispbread	2	15 g/½ oz	50/210

VEGETABLES

Many vegetables contain very little carbohydrate or calories. An average helping of any of those listed below will not add more than approximately 5 grams carbohydrate and 20–25 kcals/80–105 kJ to your diet and therefore *do not have to be counted into your diet*:

Artichokes, asparagus, aubergine, beans (runner), beansprouts, broccoli, brussels sprouts, cabbage, carrots, cauliflower, celery, courgettes, cucumber, leeks, lettuce, marrow, mushrooms, mustard and cress, okra (raw), peas (fresh or frozen), peppers, pumpkin, radishes, spinach, spring onions, swede, tomatoes (raw and canned), turnip, watercress.

Some vegetables do need to be 'counted' and those that do are listed below:

VEGETABLES	Approximate measure	Approximate weight of food in g/oz containing 10 g CHO	kcals/kJ content
* Beans, baked	60 ml/4 tbsp	75 g/3 oz	55/230
* Beans, broad, boiled	150 ml/10 tbsp	150 g/5½ oz	75/315
* Beans, dried, all types, raw	30 ml/2 tbsp	20 g/⅔ oz	55/230
Beetroot, cooked, whole	2 small	100 g/4 oz	45/190
* Lentils, dry, raw	30 ml/2 tbsp	20 g/⅔ oz	60/250
Parsnips, raw	1 small	90 g/3¼ oz	45/190
* Peas, marrow fat or processed	105 ml/7 tbsp	75 g/3 oz	60/250
* Peas, dried, all types, raw	30 ml/2 tbsp	20 g/⅔ oz	60/250
Plaintain, green, raw, peeled	small slice	35 g/1¼ oz	40/165
Potatoes, raw	1 small egg-sized	50 g/2 oz	45/190
Potatoes, boiled	1 small egg-sized	50 g/2 oz	40/165
Potatoes, chips (weighed when cooked)	4–5 av chips	25 g/1 oz	65/270
* Potatoes, jacket (weighed with skin)	1 small	50 g/2 oz	45/190
Potatoes, mashed	1 small scoop	50 g/2 oz	80/335
Potatoes, roast	½ medium	40 g/1½ oz	65/270
* Sweetcorn, canned or frozen	75 ml/5 tbsp	60 g/2 oz	45/190
* Sweetcorn, on the cob	½ medium cob	75 g/3 oz	60/250
Sweet potato, raw, peeled	1 small slice	50 g/2 oz	45/190

FRUITS

A few fruits contain very little natural sugar and can be taken in generous helpings without counting, e.g. cranberries, gooseberries, lemons, loganberries and rhubarb—all other fruits should be counted into your diet.

FRUITS	Approximate measure	Approximate weight of food in g/oz containing 10 g CHO	kcals/kJ content
Apples, eating, whole	1 medium	110 g/4 oz	50/210
Apples, cooking, whole	1 medium	125 g/4½ oz	55/230
Apples, stewed without sugar	90 ml/6 tbsp	125 g/4½ oz	40/165
Apricots, fresh, whole	3 medium	160 g/5½ oz	40/165
Apricots, dried, raw	4 small	25 g/1 oz	45/190
Bananas, with skin	14 cm/5½ inch length	90 g/3½ oz	40/165
Bananas, peeled	9 cm/3½ inch length	50 g/2 oz	40/165
Bilberries, raw	75 ml/5 tbsp	75 g/3 oz	40/165
Blackberries, raw	150 ml/10 tbsp	150 g/5½ oz	45/190
Blackcurrants, raw	150 ml/10 tbsp	150 g/5½ oz	45/190
Cherries, fresh, whole	12	100 g/4 oz	40/165
Currants, dried	30 ml/2 tbsp	15 g/½ oz	35/145
Damsons, raw, whole	7	120 g/4¼ oz	40/165
Dates, fresh, whole	3 medium	50 g/2 oz	40/165
Dates, dried, without stones	3 small	15 g/½ oz	40/165
Figs, fresh, whole	1	100 g/4 oz	40/165
Figs, dried	1	20 g/⅔ oz	40/165
Grapes, whole	10 large	75 g/3 oz	40/165
Grapefruit, whole	1 very large	400 g/14 oz	45/190
Greengages, fresh, whole	5	90 g/3¼ oz	40/165
Guavas, fresh, flesh only	1	70 g/2½ oz	45/190
Mango, fresh, whole	⅓ of a large one	100 g/4 oz	40/165
Melon, all types, weighed with skin	large slice	300 g/10½ oz	40/165
Nectarine, fresh, whole	1	90 g/3¼ oz	40/165
Orange, fresh, whole	1 large	150 g/5½ oz	40/165
Paw-paw, fresh, whole	⅙ of a large one	80 g/3 oz	50/210
Peach, fresh, whole	1 large	125 g/4½ oz	40/165
Pears, fresh, whole	1 large	130 g/4½ oz	40/165
Pineapple, fresh, no skin or core	1 thick slice	90 g/3¼ oz	40/165
Plums, cooking, fresh, whole	4 medium	180 g/6½ oz	40/165
Plums, dessert, fresh, whole	2 large	110 g/4 oz	40/165
Pomegranate, fresh, whole	1 small	110 g/4 oz	40/165
Prunes, dried, without stones	2 large	25 g/1 oz	40/165
Raisins, dried	30 ml/2 tbsp	15 g/½ oz	35/145
Raspberries, fresh	180 ml/12 tbsp	175 g/6 oz	45/190
Strawberries, fresh	15 medium	160 g/5½ oz	40/165
Sultanas, dried	30 ml/2 tbsp	15 g/½ oz	40/165
Tangerines, fresh, whole	2 large	175 g/6 oz	40/165

The amounts below provide approximately 10 grams of carbohydrate.

FRUIT JUICES	Approximate measure	Approximate weight of food in g/oz containing 10 g CHO	kcals/kJ content
Apple juice, unsweetened	90 ml/6 tbsp	85 g/3 oz	40/165
Blackcurrant juice, unsweetened	105 ml/7 tbsp	100 g/4 oz	40/165
Grapefruit juice, unsweetened	120 ml/8 tbsp	125 g/4½ oz	45/190
Orange juice, unsweetened	105 ml/7 tbsp	100 g/4 oz	40/165
Pineapple juice, unsweetened	90 ml/6 tbsp	85 g/3 oz	40/165
Tomato juice, unsweetened	1 large glass	275 g/10 oz	50/210

MILK AND MILK PRODUCTS	Approximate measure	Approximate weight of food in g/oz containing 10 g CHO	kcals/kJ content
Milk, fresh	1 cup	200 g/7 oz	130/545
Milk, fresh, skimmed	1 cup	200 g/7 oz	70/290
Milk, dried, whole	40 ml/8 tsp	25 g/1 oz	125/525
Milk, dried, skimmed	50 ml/10 tsp	20 g/⅔ oz	70/290
Milk, evaporated	90 ml/6 tbsp	90 g/3¼ oz	145/605
Yogurt, plain	1 small carton	150 g/5½ oz	80/335

ALCOHOLIC DRINKS

WINES AND BEERS	CHO value	kcals
Dry sherries	0	33 per 25 ml/1 fl oz
Dry white wine	0	18 per 25 ml/1 fl oz
Dry red wine	0	10 per 25 ml/1 fl oz
Port, ruby	3.25 g	43 per 25 ml/1 fl oz
Dry cider	10 g	150 per 450 ml/¾ pint
Vintage cider	10 g	140 per 150 ml/¼ pint
Beer, bitter, bottled	10 g	135 per 300 ml/½ pint
Beer, bitter, draught	10 g	135 per 450 ml/¾ pint
Stout, bottled	10 g	100 per 300 ml/½ pint
Diat lager	2 g	78 per 300 ml/½ pint
Ordinary lager	5 g	76 per 300 ml/½ pint

SPIRITS	CHO value	kcals
Brandy	0	63 per 25 ml/1 fl oz
Whisky	0	63 per 25 ml/1 fl oz
Gin	0	63 per 25 ml/1 fl oz
Rum	0	63 per 25 ml/1 fl oz
Vodka	0	63 per 25 ml/1 fl oz

MANUFACTURED FOODS

The foods listed below are high in sugar, and they therefore should not be used except during times of illness or in emergencies, i.e. hypos etc.

	Approximate measure	Approximate weight of food in g/oz containing 10 g CHO	kcals/kJ content
Marmalade/Jam/Honey	10 ml/2 tsp	15 g/½ oz	40/165
Lemon curd	15 ml/1 tbsp	15 g/½ oz	45/165
Golden syrup	15 ml/1 tbsp	15 g/½ oz	40/165
Black treacle	15 ml/1 tbsp	15 g/½ oz	40/165
Sugar	10 ml/2 tsp	10 g/⅓ oz	40/165
Glucose	10 ml/2 tsp	10 g/⅓ oz	40/165
Glucose tablets	3 tablets	—	40/165

The foods listed below contain a negligible amount of carbohydrate. However, their calorie content must not be forgotten when planning your meals.

	Approximate measure	Approximate weight of food in g/oz containing 10 g CHO	kcals/kJ content
Butter/Margarine	—	25 g/1 oz	185/775
Low fat spreads	—	25 g/1 oz	95/395
Egg, medium, uncooked	1	55 g/2 oz	80/335
Oil, vegetable	15 ml/1 tbsp	15 g/½ oz	135/565
Suet, shredded	90 ml/6 tbsp	50 g/2 oz	420/1755
Cream, single	small pot	150 g/5½ oz	320/1340
Cream, double	small pot	150 g/5½ oz	670/2805
Cream, whipped	small pot	150 g/5½ oz	500/2090
CHEESE			
Cheddar	small matchbox size	25 g/1 oz	100/420
Cottage	75 ml/5 tbsp	100 g/4 oz	110/460
Cream	20 ml/1 good tbsp	25 g/1 oz	110/460
Edam	small matchbox size	25 g/1 oz	75/310
Parmesan	45 ml/3 tbsp	25 g/1 oz	100/420
Stilton	small matchbox size	25 g/1 oz	115/480
Spread	45 ml/3 tbsp	50 g/2 oz	140/585
MEAT AND FISH			
Bacon, lean, grilled	1 rasher	25 g/1 oz	75/310
Bacon, lean, fried	1 rasher	25 g/1 oz	85/355
Bacon, streaky, grilled	1 rasher	25 g/1 oz	105/440
Bacon, streaky, fried	1 rasher	25 g/1 oz	125/525
Meat, lean, raw	1 av helping	100 g/3½ oz	125/540
Meat, lean, cooked	1 av helping	100 g/3½ oz	160/670
Meat, fatty, raw	1 av helping	100 g/3½ oz	410/1715
Poultry, white meat, cooked	1 av helping	100 g/3½ oz	140/585
Poultry, dark meat, cooked	1 av helping	100 g/3½ oz	155/650
Lamb cutlet, grilled	1 medium	100 g/3½ oz	250/1045
Pork chop, grilled	1 medium	150 g/5½ oz	390/1520
Corned beef	2 slices	50 g/1¾ oz	110/460

	Approximate measure	Approximate weight of food in g/oz containing 10 g CHO	kcals/kJ content
Fish fillets, white, raw	1 av helping	100 g/3½ oz	80/335
Fish fillets, fatty, raw	1 av helping	100 g/3½ oz	230/960
Shellfish, shelled	1 av helping	100 g/3½ oz	80–100/335–420
N U T S			
Almond, shelled	60 ml/4 tbsp	50 g/1¾ oz	280/1170
Brazil, shelled	14 medium	50 g/1¾ oz	310/1295
Hazelnuts, shelled	90 ml/6 tbsp	50 g/1¾ oz	190/3610
Coconut, dried	75 ml/5 tbsp	25 g/1 oz	150/625
Peanuts, roast	1 small packet	25 g/1 oz	145/605
Walnuts	16 halves	50 g/1¾ oz	130/545

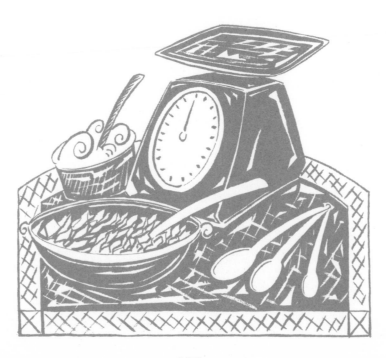

INDEX